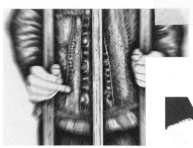

Prison Nursing

EDITED BY

ANN E. NORMAN, SEN, RGN

AND

ALAN A. PARRISH, OBE, RGN, RLND

Blackwell
Science

© 2002 by Blackwell Science Ltd,
a Blackwell Publishing Company
Editorial Offices:
Osney Mead, Oxford OX2 0EL, UK
   Tel: +44 (0)1865 206206
Blackwell Science, Inc., 350 Main Street, Malden,
MA 02148-5018, USA
   Tel: +1 781 388 8250
Iowa State Press, a Blackwell Publishing Company,
2121 State Avenue, Ames, Iowa 50014-8300, USA
   Tel: +1 515 292 0140
Blackwell Science Asia Pty Ltd, 550 Swanston Street,
Carlton South, Melbourne, Victoria 3053, Australia
   Tel: +61 (0)3 9347 0300
Blackwell Wissenschafts Verlag, Kurfürstendamm
57, 10707 Berlin, Germany
   Tel: +49 (0)30 32 79 060

First published 2002 by Blackwell Science Ltd

Library of Congress
Cataloging-in-Publication Data
is available

ISBN 0-632-05501-4

A catalogue record for this title is available from the
British Library

Set in 11/14pt Sabon
by Bookcraft Ltd, Stroud, Gloucestershire
Printed and bound in Great Britain by
TJ International, Padstow, Cornwall

For further information on
Blackwell Science, visit our website:
www.blackwell-science.com

To Teresa and Peter, my parents, who have always supported me in my chosen profession and who have helped me to balance the joys of being a parent with achieving a career that gives me so much pleasure.

My father would have been proud to have seen this book published had he still been alive.

And to all prison nursing staff: be creative, be positive, be proud!

Annie Norman

Contents

Acknowledgements   vi
Contributors   vii
Abbreviations   xi
Preface   xiii

1 The Context of Prison Nursing   1
   RHODA McCAUSLAND AND ALAN A. PARRISH

2 The Role of the Nurse in Prison Healthcare   14
   ANN E. NORMAN AND ALAN A. PARRISH

3 Prison Health: Policy Development   27
   LINDSAY BATES AND LES STOREY

4 Understanding and Changing the Dynamics of the Prison Culture   45
   SALLY THOMSON AND ALAN A. PARRISH

5 Enhancing Practice through Education   58
   SALLY THOMSON

6 Educational Developments of the Nursing Team   75
   LES STOREY

7 Legal Issues for Professional Practice   96
   MADDIE BLACKBURN

8 Quality Healthcare: Inspectorate Issues   118
   MAGGI LYNE

9 Opportunistic Healthcare: A Governor's Perspective   135
   RANNOCH DALY

10 A Reflective View   178
   STEPHEN GANNON

   Index   191

Acknowledgements

We would like to thank the editorial staff at Blackwell Science, especially Antonia Seymour, firstly for agreeing to publish the book and secondly for being so supportive and helpful through its early stages.

We owe particular thanks to Joan Hodsdon, Project Manager at Bookcraft, and her colleagues, especially Elma Burton who was kindness personified in helping us through the final stages prior to publication.

We both recognise that the book could not have been completed without the help, guidance and goodwill of Sally Thomson, and we are more than grateful to her.

Finally, we say a big thank you to the contributors to the individual chapters, without whom there could not have been a book.

Note

In April 2002 the UKCC was replaced by a new regulatory body, the Nursing and Midwifery Council. Based at the same building as the UKCC its address is: 23 Portland Place, London, W1B 1PZ (Tel: 020 7333 6697; Fax: 020 7333 6698; Website: www.nmc-uk.org).

The NMC's first action was to produce a *Code of Professional Conduct*, which became effective from 1 June 2002.

Contributors

Lindsay Bates
RGN, DN, MBA, Director of Nursing, Prison Health Policy Unit/Task Force (England and Wales)

Lindsay trained as a general nurse in the mid 1970s. She worked as a district nurse in the early to mid 1980s before moving into nursing and general management in the NHS. Lindsay worked as a hospital manager in the independent sector from 1991 to 1994 before returning to the NHS as a director of nursing for a community and mental health NHS trust in north London and subsequently an acute NHS trust. Lindsay was seconded to HM Prison Service from 1999 to 2000 as Nurse Advisor and was appointed as Director of Nursing, Prison Health Policy Unit/Task Force from July 2000. She is responsible for nursing issues, dentistry, workforce development issues (including professions allied to medicine (PAMs), and new technologies.

Maddie Blackburn
RGN, RM, Dip HV CERT, HED, MSc, Grad Dip Law

Prior to joining the Commission for Health Improvement (CHI) as a clinical governance review manager in December 2000, Maddie was the Children's Policy Officer at the Law Society. She has advised solicitors on issues relating to children and young people, drafted amendments for parliamentary bills and responded to government consultation on behalf of the Law Society. Between 1997 and 2000, Maddie was a trainee then practising solicitor specialising in claimant and defendant law; this included personal injury, NHS litigation, childcare, mental health and regulation law. Maddie regularly speaks at conferences in Britain and at international events on childcare issues, consent, confidentiality, mental capacity, human rights and the Data Protection Act. Maddie is a qualified nurse, midwife and health visitor and obtained her MSc for her work on sexuality, disability and the law. In 1998 Maddie was a specialist health visitor to HMP Holloway. She has had a number of texts published related to her work and is currently the joint editor of the RCN's child protection newsletter. She is a member of several learned societies and serves on the British Paediatric Surgeons Ethics Committee, International Research Society for Spina Bifida and /or Hydrocephalus and the RCN's Child Protection Forum Executive.

Rannoch Daly
BA in Business and Administration

Rannoch joined the prison service as an assistant governor in 1972. He worked with young offenders and adults, in high security and open prisons and at Prison Service Headquarters in the Human Resources Directorate. He was appointed Governor of HMP Hull in 1990 and HMP Leeds in 1997. He joined the Prison Health Task Force in June 2000 and has been responsible for reception screening and information management.

Stephen Gannon
RMN, RGN, MBE

Stephen trained as an RMN in Napsbury Hospital, St Albans, in the mid 1970s and later as an RGN at Central Middlesex Hospital in 1985. When asked what was the best job he's had, he said that it was as a charge nurse on the wards for nearly eight years. More an ancient mariner than a 'modern matron'! Two ENB courses, a diploma in management studies, an incomplete Master's dissertation and a Royal Yachting Association day skipper qualification later, he found a berth in the prison service in 1994. Stephen was the first chair of the Royal College of Nursing's Prison Nursing Forum and consistently rattled the chains until the fettles broke in 1998. He helped his family to found a successful private residential home and can be found occasionally wandering through a reception area near you. Stephen maintains an active interest in the Royal College of Nursing's Prison Nursing Forum as its newsletter editor. His ambition is to cruise the Caribbean in his own boat (not his current Enterprise dingy!). He was created an MBE by Her Majesty in the Millennium Honours in recognition of his work for prison nurses and received a career special recognition award from the *Nursing Standard* in 2000.

Maggi Lyne
RGN, Nursing Inspector, HM Inspectorate of Prisons 1993–2000

Maggi had an impressive career in the NHS which culminated in her becoming the Chief Nursing Officer for Ealing Health Authority. She was renowned for her creative, innovative and no-nonsense style of management. She moved from the NHS to join Her Majesty's Inspectorate of Prisons for Health Care.

Rhoda McCausland
BEd (Hons), Cert Ed (FE), RGN, RM, HV, FWT, HV Tutor and Professional Advisor

Rhoda lectured in health visiting/community nursing at the University of Ulster before taking up the post of Professional Advisor for Community Nursing/ Higher Education at the Northern Ireland National Board for Nursing, Midwifery and Health Visiting. She was deeply involved in the development of specialist practice in Northern Ireland during her time at the Board. Since early retirement she has maintained a keen interest in the continued development of the profession. Rhoda worked closely with Alan Parrish in his time as RCN Professional Officer for Prison Nursing and was particularly helpful in identifying the skill base of the nurse working in the prison environment.

Ann E. Norman
SEN, RGN, Specialist Practitioner – Practice Nursing; Assistant Director of Nursing, Prison Health Task Force (England and Wales)

Ann trained in Southampton in the 1970s. She developed her career in community nursing in the mid to late 1980s. Ann joined the prison service in 1995 at HMP Winchester, where she developed services for female prisoners. This service development gained her *Nursing Standard*'s 'Community Nurse of the Year' award in 1998 for her pioneering work. In 1998 Ann became Lead Nurse at Winchester and was recognised by the prison service in 1999 with a 'Celebrating Success' award for her achievements in prisoner healthcare. Ann was chair of the Royal College of Nursing's Prison Nursing Forum between 1998 and 2000. She moved to the Prison Health Task Force as Assistant Director of Nursing in 2001.

Alan A. Parrish
OBE, RGN, RLND, Independent Nurse Consultant and Writer

Alan was Deputy Head of Nursing Services at Harperbury Hospital in 1969. In 1972 he became Principal Nursing Officer in Leicestershire, with a countywide remit. Appointed Director of Nursing at St Lawrence's Hospital, Caterham, Surrey, Alan has also edited a book on mental handicap. He is currently writing another book in this area of practice which is due to be published in 2002. Alan became the first Nurse Advisor for Learning Disabilities at the Royal College of Nursing in 1983 and later the first Advisor for Prison Nursing at the College. He was awarded the OBE in 1999. Alan is a prolific writer of articles that highlight disadvantaged and disenfranchised groups of patients. He is well respected in the nursing profession.

Les Storey
RGN, FRCN, MSc, PG Dip HE, DMS, Dip Training Management

Les qualified in 1970 and spent over 14 years in operating theatres before moving into education and training. Les has been involved in research and development and was involved in the UKCC *Nursing in Secure Environments Project*. In October 2000 Les was awarded a Fellowship of the Royal College of Nursing in recognition of his work in relation to competence-based education and training in nursing. He was appointed to the Prison Health Policy Unit as Nursing in Prisons Occupational Standards Advisor. He was seconded from the University of Central Lancashire where he is a senior lecturer in the Faculty of Health. Les has provided advice about the development of an infrastructure to support the introduction of NVQ in custodial healthcare.

Sally Thomson
MA (Ed), BEd (Hons), RGN, RMN, RCNY, Dip N Ed, Dip N, Director of Nursing Policy and Practice, Royal College of Nursing, London

Sally's career spans both acute general and mental health nursing, with a balanced experience in both pre- and post-registration. Most of Sally's experience was at Guy's Hospital where she went on to become a nurse teacher working with pre-registration students and then post-basic and continuing education students. Sally then moved to the Royal College of Nursing where she taught psychology and education to nurse teaching students, before moving into the education policy arena. Since then Sally has been acting as Director to the professional nursing department but has retained significant links with nurse education. Sally is passionate about the development of individuals and the effect that learning geared to individual, personal and professional needs can have on a nurse's development.

Abbreviations

CBT	cognitive behavioural therapy
CHI	Commission for Health Improvement
CMG	change management group
CMHT	Community Mental Health Team
CPA	care programme approach
CPD	continuing professional development
CPT	European Committee for the Prevention of Torture and Other Inhuman and Degrading Treatment of Prisoners
ECHR	European Convention on Human Rights
ENB	English National Board
GNC	General Nursing Council
GRC	General Research Council
HAC	Health Advisory Committee
HCC	Health Care Centre
HCO	Health Care Officer
HCPO	Health Care Principal Officer
HCSO	Health Care Senior Officer
HLP	higher level of practice
HMIP	Her Majesty's Inspector of Prisons
HMP	Her Majesty's Prison
HMCIP	Her Majesty's Chief Inspector of Prisons
HNA	health needs assessment
IMR	inmate medical record
IRA	Irish Republican Army
MO	Medical Officer
NICE	National Institute for Clinical Excellence
NMC	Nursing and Midwifery Council
NSF	National Service Framework
NTO	National Training Organisation

NVQ	National Vocational Qualification
OCU	observation and classification unit
PCG	primary care group
PCT	primary care trust
PER	prisoner escort record
PHPU/TF	Prison Health Policy Unit/Task Force
POA	Prison Officers' Association
PREP	post-registration, education and practice
PSI	psychosocial intervention
RCN	Royal College of Nursing
RGN	Registered General Nurse
RMN	Registered Mental Nurse
SMO	Senior Medical Officer
S/NVQ	Scottish/National Vocational Qualificaton
UKCC	United Kingdom Central Council for Nursing, Midwifery and Health Visiting
YOI	young offenders institution

Preface

The idea for this book was very much a joint one between us, and came from our experience when we were writing articles for nursing journals in the winter of 1998. The decision to write for nursing journals about prison nurses and nursing was made by members of the Royal College of Nursing's Prison Nursing Forum, who were very unhappy about the lack of identity and appreciation of the value of nurses working in this area of care. It was during the preparation and writing of these articles that it became apparent that there was a dearth of both books and articles specifically on the role of the nurse in prison healthcare. The prison service has come under scrutiny in recent years, and has received much publicity, both adverse and positive. The service is entrenched in tradition, with an environment and culture that can be hard for an outsider to understand. The regular reports of HM Chief Inspector of Prisons, critical programmes on the television and reports in newspapers have led to changes, culminating in the publication of the joint NHS/Prison Service report *The Future Organisation of Prison Health Care* (DOH, 1999) and the more recent *Nursing in Prisons* report (DOH, 2000). Significantly for prison healthcare services this has resulted in a partnership arrangement with the NHS in an attempt to provide healthcare to prisoners equivalent to that offered to people in the wider community. This has always been an aim of the prison service but sadly one that had not been achieved previously.

Making changes

Change in any service is likely to bring about anxiety for staff, and healthcare staff in prisons are no exception. Reviewing, adjusting and changing one's attitudes is not easy on a personal basis but, with the revision of patient care services and managerial practice, it is to be hoped that services will, in the future, improve and match those of the best NHS practice.

Staff, who for years had provided a service, rightly felt threatened at the thought of working alongside colleagues from other local services who had been given the opportunity to be professionally aware and up to date on current practices. Justifiably, they also had concerns about the introduction of a change in the balance in the workforce, with a positive move to attract more nurses into prison healthcare. With this background in mind, a nursing service had to be developed and the individual nurse's role established in a primary healthcare setting that is organised and delivered within a multi-disciplinary model. Existing staff need to be convinced that there is a valued role for nurses and that they can contribute to the multi-disciplinary team.

Nurses in this area of practice have had to adapt to the environmental, cultural and bureaucratic challenges of prison life. There is an urgent need to establish credibility by producing up-to-date research that underpins and supports the value of the nurse's work. Practice needs to be scrutinised and kept under constant review, and prison nurses are professionally accountable for their practice to the Nursing and Midwifery Council (NMC). Nurses need to ensure that they have appropriate and ongoing professional updating within the guidelines set by the UKCC.

The prison nurse is not only a 'hands on' practitioner but also highlights the needs of his/her patients to a wider audience. This audience may not always be sympathetic to those needs and many will not understand the complexity of the prison population. Prisoners are from all social groups and from a range of ethnic backgrounds and ages. It seems obvious but nevertheless necessary to state that the population is transient and contains reluctant residents, who are not typical of the community whence they came in terms of the use of healthcare services. Many have not registered with a general practitioner, many have abused drugs or alcohol and many suffer from chronic diseases.

We feel that this book will help not only nurses, but many of their colleagues, who, given a team approach and partnership arrangements with the NHS, can bring about positive change in the provision of healthcare in prisons.

Ann E. Norman and Alan A. Parrish
Southampton, May 2002

References

DOH (1999) *The Future Organisation of Prison Health Care.* Report by the Joint Prison Service and National Health Service Executive Working Group. Department of Health, London.

DOH (2000) *Nursing in Prisons.* Report by the Joint Prison Service and National Health Service Executive Working Group. Department of Health, London.

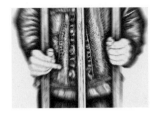

1 The Context of Prison Nursing

RHODA McCAUSLAND AND ALAN A. PARRISH

This chapter examines the social context of prison nursing, explores the principles underpinning prison nursing practice, and makes recommendations for the integration of the key skills required for specialist nursing practice.

Introduction

The practice of nursing within the setting of a prison healthcare service is at a specialist level, reflecting the uniqueness and diversity of the community it serves. Research of the literature on prison nursing in the United Kingdom soon revealed a dearth of writing about basic principles underpinning this specialist area of practice. There are publications written by other professionals about prison healthcare, but they tend to lack detail in the implementation of nursing practice. For the effective and efficient delivery of health and nursing care within the community that the prison serves, we would suggest that the principles that underpin the practice of community nursing (DHSS, 1996) be adopted as the basis of the practice of prison nursing.

In 1991 the UKCC, in its proposal for the reform of community nurse education and practice, adopted the Principles of Health Visiting for all community healthcare nurses (CETHV, 1997). The National Health Service Management Executive endorsed the principles in 1992 (NHSME, 1992).

The principles are as follows:

- the search for recognised and unrecognised health and social needs
- the prevention of ill health

- the facilitation of health-enhancing activities
- the use of therapeutic approaches to health and social care
- influencing policies affecting health and social care.

The registered nurse, equipped with the skills and knowledge acquired during general nurse training for the professional practice of nursing, will require further education and training to transfer previous knowledge and skills and develop them to a higher level of practice for this new and unique environment (Twin *et al.*, 1996).

The UKCC document *The Future of Professional Practice – The Council's Standards for Education and Practice following Registration* (UKCC, 1994), now superseded by *Standards for Specialist Education and Practice* (UKCC, 2001), clearly lays down the foundation for specialist practice, and it is within these parameters that the practice of prison nursing should be developed.

The social context of prison nursing

The ability of registered nurses to apply sociological concepts learned during training will be of paramount importance for the delivery of care within the new and more diverse environment of the prison service. The diversity of backgrounds of prisoners means that health and social needs must be assessed on an individual basis.

While the prison system treats all prisoners as equals within the category under which they have been classified, nurses must consider prisoners who come within their care with unconditional positive regard if their health needs are to be met. This will require the nurse to examine the prisoner's background in terms of class, gender, ethnicity and cultural norms and, in partnership with each prisoner, to draw up a realistic plan of care to meet identified needs.

Category A

High security prisons are recognised as being the environment for people who have committed serious criminal offences and whose escape would be highly dangerous to the public and the police, or to the security of the state.

In order to assess and meet the health needs of such prisoners the nurse has to be aware of the social class and strata from which they have come. Their needs will be highly diverse, as prisoners come from all social strata. The nurse practising in this setting will be exposed to a much higher level of risk and stress because of the rigidity of the top security regime required to hold these prisoners in custody. Good team management will depend on the interaction between the nursing team and the prison service, as well as the leadership skills available within that team. A thorough understanding of the role of the prison governor and prison officers is essential for the effective and efficient service necessary for good client care.

For nurses to practise within the law it is important that they understand the policies that underpin the functioning of a prison. The necessity of the nurse to practise and function within the limits set out in the *The Scope of Professional Practice* (UKCC, 1992) must be acknowledged. It is essential that professional supervision is available for the nurse and partnership arrangements with local NHS providers will enhance and enrich this as well as making its facilitation easier. The delivery of healthcare of a defined and acceptable quality will and does depend on the co-operation, respect and goodwill of all personnel working within this high security environment.

Category B

This category applies to those prisoners for whom the very highest conditions of security are not necessary but for whom escape must be made very difficult. Unsentenced prisoners are automatically categorised B unless they are provisionally placed in Category A. The application of sociological concepts, however, is still required to ensure the delivery of efficient and effective healthcare. The nurse is less exposed to the very rigid practices of a high security environment although security and custody must always be the top priority in any prison. The delivery of healthcare can be considered at a different level and programmes of health education and healthy lifestyles introduced more easily. Prison policies still apply: security and custody remain the priority. The registered nurse must always be aware of the need to comply with the UKCC/NMC rules (UKCC, 1992).

Category C

Prisoners who cannot be placed in open conditions but who do not have the ability, resources or the will to make an escape attempt come into Category C. Many Category C prisons will be there primarily for training of the prisoners.

Category D

Category D prisoners can be reasonably trusted to serve their sentences in open conditions. Many of these prisoners will be nearing a release date from prison and often work on a daily basis in the local community.

Women's prisons

The physical environment of a women's prison differs very little from that of a men's prison in both the high and low security establishments. The challenge of providing good quality healthcare equivalent to that of the local NHS is an ongoing struggle for the multi-disciplinary team. The complexity of the relationships between the professionals and the clients is amplified within this environment. This is doubly so when women are in a system that is designed for men, and although there have been marked improvements in the environment over the years, it is still lacking in some of the finer requirements for a woman in custody. The Chief Inspector of Prisons points out (Home Office, 1997) that

> The multiple and severe health problems experienced by many women who become prisoners are made more profound by personal and family history, sexual and physical abuse, their role as carers, the stress of imprisonment, isolation and drug dependence.

The health needs of women are significantly different from those of men and many women who enter prison come from socially disadvantaged backgrounds. This often means that they have poor health and a far greater exposure to risk behaviour than other women and this puts their overall health status at risk. They are also ignorant of, or reluctant to discuss or disclose, their personal health problems. Some of these women live on the margins of the healthcare system, with greater than average health problems (often very numerous and complex) because of the situations in which they find themselves. These problems can be because of malnutrition, sexual abuse by a number of partners, poor housing or the manifestations of living life at a very high level of stress.

It is because of the complex and often painful background from which some of these women have come that sensitivity is needed when trying to provide a service equivalent to that of the NHS outside the prison environment. Because of their past experiences, it is a priority to ensure that these women have a choice of being seen by a female doctor and treated wherever possible by a female nurse, if that is their wish.

It is also crucial to take the opportunity, while a woman is in prison, to give her a proper health assessment and expose her to health education and health promotion facilities. While serving a sentence in prison women should benefit from all the actions that are taken to improve the health of the whole nation. Women prisoners often miss out on some of the positive advances that take place in the community in respect of women's health, either because of their circumstances or because, for whatever reason, they do not feel able to take advantage of the chances on offer. Examples of services that are often missed are cervical screening and mammography.

The importance of implementing present healthcare policies regarding women's health should be and is being encouraged through the partnership arrangements with the NHS. The establishment of a Women's Policy Unit has shown that the prison service recognises the special needs of women and has a commitment to meeting those needs.

Men in prison

Men make up the majority of people who are held in prison, across an age range of 15 years to over 80 years. Within this group there is a wide range of ethnic, cultural and gender specific issues, and attitudes towards health. Among some of the most important issues are substance abuse, attitudes towards sex, and sexual practices, along with some macho-style behaviours that are often a front or a cover for an insecure person. Men are less likely to access health services than women and, therefore, greater emphasis needs to be placed on the role of the nurse in prison to provide opportunities for men to be exposed to both health education and health promotion activities. This needs to be done creatively, subtly and in a personalised manner.

It is becoming increasingly the norm in healthcare centres for men's health clinics (Well Man Clinics) to be organised on a regular basis. It is here that the real issues around an individual's health are identified and suitable treatments arranged. Within the prison setting the nurse will need to set up health promotion activities to meet identified needs, for example, screening for heart disease, and testicular and prostate cancer. Setting up such clinics may also have the effect of triggering health awareness issues for male staff. It is to be hoped that the partnership arrangements with the local national health services will eventually bring about the introduction of good quality occupational health services for all staff working in a prison environment.

Young offenders institutions

A young offender is defined as someone who is between 15 and 21 years of age.

The environment provided for young offenders is varied because of the diverse nature and age of the population that it serves. Such units vary in terms of the facilities for the young offender and the regimes that are organised. For example, Lancaster Farms, in Lancashire, is self-contained, with an emphasis on outdoor pursuits within the confines of the institution. The nurse practising in this setting will need to have the ability to apply both sociological and psychological concepts to this group who have particular and special needs at this crucial time in their lives. A specialist knowledge of adolescence and family dynamics will be required for the nurse to understand and provide the level of care that is needed for this vulnerable group of offenders.

The influence of policies affecting the health of this group will be of paramount importance: for example, health screening, smoking, masochistic behaviour, sexual practices, anger management therapy, etc. These young people are often emotionally vulnerable and a staff member is commonly seen as a role model; staff need to respect the significance and importance of this.

If there is to be any real success, effective teamwork is essential, involving all the professionals working within the prison to deliver the level of care required both for primary care and to prepare for rehabilitation back into the community.

Detention centres

These centres are run by the prison service for the holding of detainees and they are the only area within the service where the crime committed by the individual is not known by the staff.

Specialist practice for prison nursing

The Future of Professional Practice – The Council's Standards for Education and Practice following Registration (UKCC, 1994) revised in *Standards for Specialist Education and Practice* (UKCC, 2001) reaffirms four broad areas of practice for the specialist nurse. Specialist practice requires higher levels of judgement, discretion and decision-making to be exercised in these areas, namely:

(1)   clinical nursing practice
(2)   care and programme management
(3)   clinical practice management
(4)   clinical practice leadership.

The higher level of practice can be exercised in any area of healthcare delivery. The standards to ensure this are set out in the document. As stated previously, the registered nurse working within the prison service setting practises at specialist level. The four broad areas identified by the *Standards for Specialist Education and Practice* (UKCC, 2001) therefore apply to the registered nurse working in the specialist area of prison nursing. In order for the prison nurse to function at this higher level of practice, appropriate programmes of education and training need to be set up that cover these four areas.

Clinical nursing practice

Clinical nursing practice aims to enhance the knowledge and skills required to meet the specialist clinical needs of the clients/patients within the care of the nurse. In this case, prisoners are being nursed in an environment not always conducive to the meeting of their particular and individual needs, and nurses are working within a restrictive and regimented environment.

Care and programme management

Care and programme management relates to individuals, their families and the environment in which they are receiving care. Co-ordination of care is the core focus. Health promotion, disease prevention, risk-taking analysis and diagnosis feature as key areas for competence development.

Clinical practice leadership

The specialist prison nurse will be expected to lead and deliver the health service in response to an individual prisoner's needs. This should equate with the standard and range of care that can be received in local national health services. The specialist prison nurse will also support and supervise nurses and other care staff within his or her particular remit of practice. Other skills will include teaching, assessment and resource management. These leadership skills will have to be practised in an environment that is governed by restrictive regimes and the need for security at all times.

Clinical practice management

This area requires specialist nurses to set, monitor and evaluate care standards and the effectiveness of their nursing actions. Prison nurses will need an in-depth knowledge of clinical practice development in their area of specialism. The need to be innovative and to use initiative should always be part of the specialist agenda in the delivery of care. Practising in prison healthcare offers nurses this opportunity albeit they have to take into account the restrictions that a prison naturally imposes on the way they practise.

Application of the principles to the practice of prison nursing

The search for health needs

This will require prison nurses to search and identify the physical, psychological, social and spiritual needs of prisoners who come within the scope of their care. It will involve an in-depth search in partnership with individuals, if their needs are to be met within the restricted regime of custodial care. The prison nurse may wish to use a theoretical framework as a guide to practice for the application of the search for health needs principle. Bradshaw's taxonomy of need (1972) is suggested, as it considers need across four dimensions – Normative, Felt, Expressed and Comparative.

Normative needs

Normative need is defined in accordance with an agreed standard laid down by an expert or professional and compared with a standard that already exists. The normative needs of prisoners will embrace the physical needs of all human beings: food, water, warmth, shelter and protection.

Whatever the nature of the crimes they may have committed, prisoners need to be considered with unconditional positive regard if their psychological and spiritual needs are to be met. These needs will differ according to the value judgements of other experts – for example, probation officers, social workers and medical staff – particularly in the areas of nutrition, exercise, rehabilitation and the maintenance of health.

There will be a norm or standard set within the different areas of custodial care. Prison nurses need to be able to question the standards set and act accordingly for the benefit of the prisoner in relation to the maintenance of health.

Felt needs

Felt needs are those identified by the individual as particular wants that need to be addressed. As felt need is limited by the perspective of the individual, prisoners may expect an unreasonable response to the meeting of such need. Because of their particular mindset they may well feel all requests to meet their needs should be granted. The prisoner may not identify unrecognised needs with regard to health, for example, the need for behaviour change in relation to drug taking, smoking and the maintenance of health in general. It is here that the health needs assessment is so important and the prisoner's involvement in that process is the key to an accurate result.

Expressed needs

Expressed needs are the demands for felt needs to be turned into actions. The meeting of these needs may be difficult for the prison nurse, as there may be conflict because of the policies and strict regime of the prison and the differing opinions of other member of the prison team.

Comparative needs

The search for comparative needs will involve the prison nurse in data collection and analysis of empirical evidence of different prison communities in order to compare and contrast how prisoners are facilitated and treated within the different settings. Comparative analyses will assist prison nurses in the influencing of policy that may affect the health of the clientele who come within their care.

Prevention of ill health

The prevention of ill health within the prison setting is of paramount importance for the maintenance of a disease-free environment and for the health of the people within that environment.

The prevention of ill health and the promotion of health may be based on Caplan's (1961) concept of three levels of prevention.

Primary prevention

Primary prevention aims at the maintenance of good health. To maintain health and prevent disease, it is essential to have a healthy environment in which to exist. There is a need to have the basic necessities to maintain health: for example, clean air, food, water, warmth, adequate living space and good sanitation.

The history of prisons in this respect is not good and many will have read of the Victorian times when the prison was not the healthiest place in which to spend time, with gross overcrowding and basic human functions done in a bucket and slopped out each morning. The prison governor has a key role to play in primary prevention by insisting that there are smoking-free zones and that healthy meals are provided, along with the opportunity for prisoners to have a reasonable amount of exercise. The prison nurse, in applying this concept to practice, has a duty to assess the environment within the different categories of custodial care. This is to ensure that the needs of prisoners are met in terms of a healthy environment, in order to prevent disease occurring and to maintain the health of the prisoner being exposed to this environment. With the growth of infectious diseases such as tuberculosis, HIV and AIDS, programmes of prevention should be provided within the regimes of the prison.

Secondary prevention

Secondary prevention concerns the early detection and treatment of disease. The prison nurse's contribution to this lies in the development of disease prevention schemes and the encouragement of prisoners to take up such schemes. Programmes of this nature may include screening for heart disease, AIDS, breast and cervical cancer, mental health issues and drug abuse. A prisoner, although segregated from the community, is entitled to equity when it comes to healthcare and the new partnership arrangements with the local national health services should go some way to ensure this is achieved.

Tertiary prevention

This is an aspect of aftercare, concerned with containing and limiting the effects of a particular condition. The nurse in prison healthcare has a duty to give and maintain the appropriate care to all prisoners, but in particular to those with chronic conditions or in long-term care or custody.

Protection of vulnerable groups

The protection of vulnerable groups within a prison setting is as important as the protection of such groups outside the prison. Vulnerable prisoners may be those who are detained for the crime they have committed but who are not hardened criminals – for example the upper-class fraudster, the person committed for assault for protecting their own property, the mentally ill, the person with a learning disability, the driver who has killed someone in a road accident. The members of a team looking after such groups of prisoners need to work closely together to protect and meet the health and social needs of these individuals in order for them to survive and be effectively and efficiently rehabilitated back into the community with their families and friends.

The level of psychiatric morbidity among prisoners is known to be much higher than that in the general population. About 75% of inpatients in prison healthcare centres have mental health problems (Reed & Lyne, 2000). There are strong recommendations in *The Future Organisation of Prison Health Care* (DOH, 1999) regarding the quality and standards of care that should be provided in the new partnership arrangements that are developing with the NHS.

- The care of mentally ill prisoners should develop in line with NHS mental health and policy and NHS frameworks including new arrangements for referral and admission to high and medium secure psychiatric services.
- Special attention should be paid to better identification of mental health needs at the reception screening.
- Mechanisms should be put in place to ensure the satisfactory functioning of a care programme approach within prisons and the development of mental health outreach work on prison wings.
- Prisoners should receive the same level of community care within prison as they would receive in the wider community, and policies should be put in place to ensure adequate and effective communication between NHS mental health services and prisons. Health authorities should ensure that service agreements with NHS trusts include appropriate mental health services for prisoners with appropriately qualified staff.

This standard of service should be the aim within every prison. If achieved it would certainly go a long way to ensuring that these particularly vulnerable prisoners were better protected and prepared for their move back into the community, where the seamless service envisaged would ensure continuity of care.

Facilitation of health-enhancing activities

In order to promote healthy lifestyles, the prison nurse will endeavour to stimulate an awareness of health needs with the clientele within the prison community. Empowering prisoners to adopt healthy lifestyles within a rigid and restrictive environment may be extremely difficult for the nurse. Tones (1991) explores the concept of empowerment and refers to it as a process whereby the individual or a community of individuals acquires power or the capacity to control other people and resources, while self-empowerment focuses on the individual's capacity to control his or her own life. Gibson (1991) sees empowerment as a process of promoting people's ability to meet their own needs, solve their own problems and mobilise the necessary resources to feel in control.

The nurse may experience difficulty empowering prisoners to adopt a healthy lifestyle, when they have little or no control over the prison regime or their lives. There is a need, therefore, to work in close partnership with the other members of the prison service, to develop action plans that will enhance the health of the prison community and to provide health-enhancing activities in response to identified needs. The rigidity of the regimes and the attitudes and perceptions of the prisoners may act as a barrier to the development of such activities.

Therapeutic approaches to health and social care

In applying this principle to the practice of prison nursing, one of the most fundamental questions the prison nurse must ask is 'Why did I choose this area of practice?' The answer to this question is the first step to self-awareness and self-monitoring (Long, 2001). Embraced within this notion is the belief that the nurse's therapeutic presence has a complex role to play in the promotion of health, healing and recovery (Slevin & Long, 2000). Nurses can act as positive role models. Prisoners experience healing when they come to accept what nurses think, say, feel and believe; this acceptance can lead prisoners to experience positive interactions that give them a sense of worth and dignity (Long, 1997). To deny prisoners such therapeutic experiences is to deny them all that is best in humanity, beginning with the premise that nurses and prisoners are equal as human beings. It is important, therefore, that all prison nurses are provided with structured opportunities to explore what the 'self' is, and what it means to be human, before reflecting on the use of 'self' as a therapeutic catalyst. This is the basis upon which the development and maintenance of the therapeutic relationship is built, regardless of which therapeutic approach to care is chosen, implemented and evaluated (Long, 2001). Furthermore, it is important that prison nurses are educated and trained to work as autonomous practitioners as well as team members who will provide a range of therapeutic approaches appropriate to meeting the needs of individual clients and clinical supervision (Cutcliff & Butterworth, 2001). A regular structured approach to the delivery of care is recommended, for example, the 40-minute period of contact per week from the first week of the prisoner's sentence. Used wisely, the results of successful scientific research can be integrated into therapeutic care to enhance and advance professional prison nursing practice. The ultimate aim is to provide best practice and high quality care and promote the health and well-being of the total prison population.

Influencing policies affecting health and social care

Prison nurses are the assessors of health needs within the prison setting. They work within the parameters of the policies set down by the Joint Prison Service and National Health Service Executive Working Group (DOH, 1999) and *The Scope of Professional Practice* (UKCC, 1992). It is their duty to implement the policies that affect the health of the clients within their care. They also act as agents of change. To do this they use the knowledge gained from the assessment and analysis of the needs within their particular prison community to influence policy change for the maintenance of good physical and mental health.

Summary

This chapter has endeavoured to consider the specialist practice of prison nursing. It has looked at the social context in which it is delivered and addressed the *Standards for Specialist Education and Practice* as defined by the UKCC/NMC (2001), outlining the broad areas for education and practice. The principles of community nursing (DHSS, 1996) have been suggested to underpin the practice of prison nursing delivered within the custodial institutions throughout the United Kingdom. The chapter concluded with suggestions as to how these principles may be applied to the practice of prison nursing.

References

Bradshaw, J. (1972) The concept of social need. *New Society*, 30, 640–3.

Caplan, G. (1961) *An Approach to Community Mental Health*. Tavistock Publications, London.

CETHV (1997) *An Investigation into the Principles and Practice of Health Visiting*. Council for the Education and Training of Health Visitors, London.

Cutcliff, J. & Butterworth, T. (2001) *Clinical Supervision*. Routledge, London.

DHSS (1996) *A Strategy for Nursing Midwifery and Health Visiting in Northern Ireland*. HMSO, Northern Ireland.

DOH (1999) *The Future Organisation of Prison Health Care*. Report by the Joint Prison Service and National Health Service Executive Working Group. Department of Health, London.

Gibson, C.H. (1991) A concept analysis of empowerment. *Journal of Advanced Nursing*, 16, 354–61.

Home Office (1997) *Women in Prison. A thematic review*. HMIP, Home Office, London.

Long, A. (2001) Mental health nursing. In: *Community Health Care Nursing*, (eds D. Sines, F. Appleby & B. Raymond). Blackwell Science, Oxford.

Long, A. (1997) Approaches to care of vulnerable groups. In: *Quality Issues in Community Health Care Nursing*, (ed. C. Mason). Macmillan, Oxford.

NHSME (1992) *Guidance on the Extension of the Hospital and Community Services. Elements of GP Fundholding Scheme, April 1993 Et48 (92)*. National Health Service Executive, London.

Reed, J. & Lyne, M. (2000) Inpatient care of the mentally ill people in prison: results of a year's programme of semi-structured inspections. *British Medical Journal*, 320, 1031–4.

Slevin, E. & Long, A. (2000) *Therapeutic Presence in Advanced Interactions in Community Health Care Nursing*. Macmillan, Oxford.

Tones, A. (1991) Health promotion empowerment and the psychology of control. *Journal of the Institute of Health Education*, 29(1), 17–26.

Twin, S., Roberts, B. & Anderson, S. (1996) *Community Health Care Nursing*. Butterworth Heinemann, London.

UKCC (1992) *The Scope of Professional Practice*. United Kingdom Central Council for Nursing, Midwifery and Health Visiting, London.

UKCC (1994) *The Future of Professional Practice – The Council's Standards for Education and Practice following Registration*. United Kingdom Central Council for Nursing, Midwifery and Health Visiting, London.

UKCC (2001) *Standards for Specialist Education and Practice*. Registrar's Letter. 11/2001. United Kingdom Central Council for Nursing, Midwifery and Health Visiting, London.

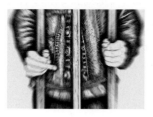

2 The Role of the Nurse in Prison Healthcare

ANN E. NORMAN AND ALAN A. PARRISH

This chapter, provided by the editors of this book, is designed to engage the reader in further debate. It has been developed following lengthy discussions with prison nurses, academics, prison staff and a whole host of interested professionals seeking to understand 'the role of the prison nurse'. Readers may have alternative views or additional issues that they would wish to raise from reading this chapter; the intention is to encourage debate in order to shape and solidify collective thinking.

Introduction

This chapter looks at the multi-faceted and specialist role of the nurse in prison healthcare. It focuses on:

- the wide range of challenges and frustrations that affect nursing practice in this unique environment
- the challenge of balancing issues relating to the provision of both custody and care that feature as a constant part of a nurse's daily life in prison
- the pivotal role of addressing and ensuring the quality of care provision, and enhancement of the standard of the healthcare service through a multi-disciplinary team approach
- the value of effective teamwork and respect for the contribution made by other members of the healthcare team.

The role of the nurse working within the prison service is multi-faceted. It embraces the assessment of the physical, psychological, emotional, spiritual and social needs of individual clients/patients in custodial care, the actual transaction of care delivery and care management, counselling, health education, collaboration with other agencies, clinical decision-making, advocacy and rehabilitation.

Prison nursing practice demands the integration of a range of key concepts that underpin the essence of nursing. These relate to the provision of psychosocial support and the application and consideration of the nurse's own professional value system. Nurses also need to develop key skills designed to encourage clients to make informed choices and decisions that will enable clients to return to independent living and maximum adaptation.

The transfer of nursing skills from a hospital or community setting to the prison setting of custodial care demands a more specialist and higher level of clinical decision-making and practice. One key issue relating to such adaptation concerns the comparatively skewed skill mix that exists in prison services for qualified nurses. This will often demand that qualified nurses extend their role and scope of professional practice to cover a significantly varied range of competences and practices. This change is both challenging and demanding and requires time for the necessary adjustments to take place. Among the challenges confronting prison healthcare nurses are the diverse nature of the area in which they practise and an increasing need to form meaningful and effective partnership arrangements with the local services in the NHS. One other key challenge has been the implementation of multi-disciplinary care delivery, associated with a more effective, efficient and flexible approach to the organisation of client care and delivery through the provision of healthcare clinics. Such developments are characteristic of the implementation of a primary care model of care delivery.

Prison nurses will also be increasingly required to demonstrate that care is effectively and responsively delivered to meet the needs of the prison population. The achievement of such an aim is an issue that healthcare managers will need to address. In so doing it will be important to prove by good quality research that nurses, through their practice and activities, make a significant impact on the health of prisoners.

Nurse–patient relationships

Prison nursing is recognised as an area where the nurse–patient relationship and its boundaries are of paramount importance. Many of the clients with whom prison nurses work may present specific challenges with regard to manipulative behaviours that can be designed to compromise and undermine the essence of nursing care. In such cases the margin of error (for the nurse) is small and may hold greater significance and accountability if things should go wrong.

Nurses who practise in prison healthcare will find this context radically different from most of their previous experience. For example, the nurse will have to deal with the delicate balance between security and care on a daily basis. Prison regimes and culture are also major contingent factors that influence the way in which nurses function and they need to assimilate this in order to deliver effective care. Prison life is – and has to be – governed by the security needs of the prison, placing everything else in a secondary position. This precept will demand immediate adoption if nurses are to demonstrate credibility both to their clients and to employers, though it may present ethical dilemmas. Compliance, conformity and socialisation are essential to the provision and maintenance of a safe environment and have to be an integral part of the lives of all who reside or work within the prison population.

The effective nurse will demonstrate to the service professionalism, experience, competence and an in-depth knowledge of both illness and the promotion of good health. These skills and attributes will be deployed within the context of a multi-disciplinary team, thus enriching care practice and collaborative care management. The ability to assess a situation, using evidence-based problem-solving, making clinical decisions and being able to act on those decisions makes for a more effective and efficient service for the client and is truly valuable in a cost-conscious era.

Prison nurses as key members of such a team have the additional responsibility of providing 24-hour care to their clients (as opposed to single episodes of care provided by other members of the care team – for example, physiotherapists). They also provide overall direction to the individual's particular healthcare needs, collaborating with the patient/client and working with other team members to ensure that an appropriate level of care is consistently delivered, monitored and evaluated. These functions have to be undertaken in the special context of the prison environment, which differs from the context in which a nurse would normally practise. Security and custody are over-riding factors in all care-giving in prison situations, and treatments must be organised around time-focused regimes that will be a new phenomenon to many nurses. The co-ordination of an individual's care is a central function of the nurse's role in the prison healthcare environment. To ensure that each patient/client receives good quality care it is essential that there is good communication between professionals and that treatment, therapies and consultations are both consistent and regularly evaluated. It is therefore essential that the system of direct communication between staff is of a suitable quality and standard to ensure continuity and uninterrupted care. Clear two-way communication and message-passing are keys to the success of this aspect of service provision. The opportunity to free up medical staff to do more appropriate work, by organising and maximising nursing skills, has led to the implementation of nurse-led clinics. (This does not preclude clients/prisoners from having the right to see a doctor.) Such clinics are commonplace in some prisons and need to be extended. Such extension of the scope of nursing practice must be accompanied by investment in the further educational development of prison nurses. New demands for enhanced knowledge and competences will call for the provision of continuous professional development and engagement in both reflective practice and clinical supervision. Engagement in such processes will ensure that prison nurses are fit for the purpose through their application of the necessary level of competence to guarantee patient safety and quality of service (benchmarked against national standards of care practice).

Nurses can make a remarkable impact on healthcare in prisons (Norman & Parrish, 1999a, b). They have influenced a wide range of care areas, but, in particular, the recruitment of registered nurses with a background and training in mental healthcare has helped to improve the quality of care for prisoners as well as giving professional support to unqualified colleagues who work alongside prison nurses in a supporting role. This contribution is recognised in the report *The Future Organisation of Prison Health Care* (DOH, 1999, p. 30, para. 65):

> Psychiatric nurses with experience of forensic setting, risk management, the management of violence and skills in therapeutic approaches such as cognitive therapy would greatly improve the care of mentally disordered offenders.

Prison nursing is varied and its practitioners range from the nurse working in public health and primary healthcare to those who work in dedicated mental health settings within the prison environment. It is the diversity of the roles of prison nurses and their pioneering work that present new challenges for practitioners and demand the application of multiple roles and competences. The ability of prison nurses to respond effectively to these challenges has ensured that they will be recognised as key players in the profession over the next decade.

Client group

The healthcare needs of prisoners are very varied and place these clients in one of the most vulnerable groups in society. Their situations are often self-inflicted by their own neglect and lifestyle. Prison nurses will therefore need to be familiar with the prisoners' idiosyncratic behaviours and be able to respond to their multiple and often unfulfilled health needs. It has been shown that imprisonment and a vigilant health assessment via nurses and their colleagues in the multi-disciplinary team can bring about a dramatic improvement in an individual's health and lifestyle. When such assessments are combined with the provision of health education and health promotion sessions, positive changes may be witnessed in both the individual's thinking and lifestyle, which will hopefully continue on return to the community and the development of a new partnership arrangement with the NHS. Such partnerships were advocated by, among others, Hancock in 1999 (Hancock, 1999). Partnership policies are now gradually becoming the norm, and prison healthcare and local NHS nurses are working together with social services and other supportive community services to ensure that prisoners receive a seamless service. At present, however, a seamless service is a rare achievement – but it is something that should be aimed for. This will mean working across all professional and organisational boundaries, involving all agencies including police, housing departments, probation and local residents groups. The provision of a community link nurse (from the local primary care trust) with the prison healthcare service will be pivotal to the success of such a service. Similarly, more progressive establishments will appoint a prison nurse to develop relationships with local service providers. This liaison person could be a positive contact for colleagues and fellow professionals and be a valuable resource ensuring the provision of a client-led quality service.

Leadership

Difficulties may be experienced in securing the inter-professional collaboration which everyone knows to be essential if the prison healthcare service is to be truly effective, efficient and of sound quality. If it is to match that of the local health service, managers at all levels in the service will need to address and promote such alliances. It is inevitable that different professionals will see things differently, but the need for positive leadership and co-operation is paramount. The other essential ingredient to multi-disciplinary working is the provision of a flexible workforce that operates within an atmosphere of openness and honesty, where role differences can be clarified, understood and valued, and new skills learned.

   Although sterling efforts have been made by a range of different categories of health staff to facilitate the provision of a quality service, the prison organisation, its internal systems and all parts of the infrastructure are geared to the primary goal of custody and effective security procedures. This philosophy and regime may militate against the provision of high quality healthcare. Consequently the delivery of effective nursing services is challenging within an organisation that is both bureaucratic and restrictive in the application of its work policies. This is compounded within a culture where new ways of working, however exciting or innovative, are sometimes regarded with suspicion. This environment does, however, provide challenges and opportunities for nurses to experience the chance to practise in a setting that is almost always different from their previous areas of work.

Over the past decade the nurse has developed an important role as catalyst in the prison healthcare system. While bringing a more humane, sensitive and individual approach to the work they do, prison nurses must balance this with the need to maintain security and custody standards in prison life. This is a position that is recognised and acknowledged by nurses and understood to be essential in respecting and protecting both themselves and colleagues.

Getting it right

In any organisation or institution, its spirit and atmosphere depend not only on the rules and regulations that are in force but also on the attitudes and personality of the staff and the leadership style. In a prison, where staff hold significant power and control over the lives of prisoners, the correct attitude and professional behaviour of staff are key determinants to a prison being well run. In such a prison staff are likely to enjoy coming to work and feel valued. This makes recruitment and selection of new staff and the ongoing training and education of existing staff vitally important to the maintenance of morale.

The penal system has its critics. Some have the view that the service is too punitive and negative, with too little emphasis on the education of prisoners and on their preparation for returning to the community. Others take the view that the balance has moved too much in favour of the criminal, and ignores the interests of the people they may have injured, abused or offended. Nurses as individuals will have different ways of dealing with this and may need to share their thoughts and views, in confidence, with another colleague or their line manager. Clinical supervision is a useful vehicle to achieve this objective.

It is most important for all staff to remember that the prisoners' sentences and exclusion from mainstream society are their punishment. Nurses will have an opinion and a view of a prisoner's offence and it may be extremely difficult not to show disapproval, but at all times professionalism must be maintained and no hint of individual feelings should be made apparent. There is no place for judgemental attitudes; it is important to be able to accept prisoners with unconditional positive regard. This may severely test the professionalism of the nurse, but it is essential that nurses maintain such standards in accordance with the UKCC/NMC *Code of Professional Conduct* (UKCC, 1992).

Challenging times ahead

The continuing success and credibility of any profession are dependent upon, among other things, its ability to respond to challenges, changes and expectations of service users and society. Nurses working in prison healthcare are facing a challenging time in the new partnership arrangements with the NHS and the changes and developments this heralds for the service over the next decade (DOH, 1999). Clearly, nurses will retain and maintain their prime position at the cutting edge of the service as these improvements and partnership arrangements with local NHS providers take place. Changes will be inevitable and necessary as the two services work through the embryonic stages of the new partnership. It is here that nurses can be the catalysts for change since they have an understanding of both the NHS and the prison service culture and of each other's roles and skills.

Nursing is noted for its ability to change, and nurses have always had a flexible approach to their work, responding well to the challenges and changes to services with the introduction of new policies. Clinical governance provides an excellent medium for the creation of a learning organisation (DOH, 2001a). Its application refers to the need to make arrangements within the service for the management, monitoring and improvement of the quality of prison healthcare and the management of risk. It is a concept already developed in the NHS and is an important part of the government's programme of modernisation.

Facing challenges, or adjusting to changes in their patterns of work, is a fairly regular occurrence for nurses generally and no nurse has to face more challenges than a nurse practising in prison healthcare. The more successful professions are those with the vision to perceive the need for self-appraisal and a flexible approach to the provision of those services for which they are responsible. Prison healthcare has developed over the years in line with the changes that have taken place in services outside the prisons, despite adverse surroundings and a difficult clientele. Progress continues to be made, and it is to be hoped that the increase in the number of nurses and the multi-disciplinary team approach in the day-to-day working of the healthcare unit will ensure that this improvement is not just maintained but increased. The old-fashioned notion of a prison as an isolated and segregated unit in the community will no longer be accepted by a society that has moved on with its thinking. The philosophy of a primary healthcare-led integrated healthcare service for all is seen by most as forward thinking and an integral part of that service should be its extension into the prison healthcare system. This in itself can only be good for the prisoners and the prison healthcare professionals alike, who daily try to meet their clients' needs in a service that often does not have either the resources or the necessary workforce available.

Poised for change

Prison nurses have been employed within a system that was out of date and over-medicalised but is now poised and ready for change. The publication of the report by the Joint Prison Service and National Health Service Executive Working Group *The Future Organisation of Prison Health Care* (DOH, 1999) outlines the direction that the service is taking and the key word throughout is partnership. The stated aim of prison healthcare is noted to be:

> To give prisoners access to the same quality and range of healthcare services as the general public receive from the National Health Service.

The chance to work closely with the local NHS in a partnership relationship is both timely and essential if the above aim is to be met. However, at present the service is not equitable across the country, either in terms of what is on offer or in quality. There is considerable variation in the links that have or have not been formed with local primary healthcare services. Making change in any organisation is difficult, however well the changes are planned, but to make changes to the life and working of a prison is a real challenge. The introduction of the partnership arrangements will inevitably bring about insecurity and anxiety in some staff and will demand that nurses adjust to the way they work in the new style of service, as it develops with the local services. It is important to emphasise that this is not likely to be a one-way process, since nurses coming into prisons for the first time will have similar anxieties and worries about how their practice will match up to that of the established prison nurse.

The introduction of the partnership arrangements with the NHS will be seen by most staff as having a positive impact on the prison healthcare service. This should be viewed as a positive development by healthcare staff. The introduction of staff to local services and the chance for staff to invite relevant and competent colleagues from a range of professions into the prisons is an exciting venture, and an opportunity not to be missed. For example, Lindsay Bates has pointed out that there will be opportunities for joint training and shared educational experiences with professional colleagues in local services (Alderman, 1999). Carrying out health needs assessments in partnership with the NHS will also enable staff from both sectors to demonstrate their individual competences and skills with the aim of facilitating their transfer between the NHS and the prison healthcare system (and *vice versa*). The outcome will be gradual development of normative standards and equality of care practice.

Both men and women from foreign countries and differing cultural or ethnic backgrounds have particular difficulties when serving a sentence in prison and these have to be respected (Richards *et al.*, 1995). Prison nurses will therefore have to take cognisance of the social and ethnic needs of the prison population. This needs to be shown in the recruitment of suitably selected staff from ethnic backgrounds similar to those of prisoners and reflecting an understanding of the cultural aspects of their lives. There is also an educational exercise to be conducted with existing staff, who, through no fault of their own, may be unaware of the customs, culture and needs of particular ethnic groups. Quite apart from the stress of their imprisonment and separation from their families, prisoners have to adjust to a range of changes and experiences in prison that would not be part of their lives in their indigenous communities.

For some there will be language difficulties, and attention needs to be given to the recruitment of staff from similar cultural backgrounds. If this not be possible, then links with local voluntary organisations should be established to ensure that effective communication, advocacy and liaison are provided. Specific cultural, religious, dietary and ethnic needs will also need specific responses. Both men and women will have particular and individual needs that have to be addressed in respect of receiving healthcare treatments the 'western way'.

For example, clients may present with feelings of shame and guilt. Alleviating these feelings through sharing them with others may not be acceptable in some cultures; not even sharing with friends and family members, let alone strangers from another culture. This need for privacy should be acknowledged and dealt with in a way that will not add to the client's stress or discomfort. Also, the more intimate procedures (such as body searches), which most people find humiliating, could be construed as rape in some cultures, so this type of procedure needs to be conducted in a very sensitive manner.

Vulnerable people

Hancock (1999) emphatically states that nurses need to work with people who feel excluded from society:

> If you are poor, black, vulnerable, mentally ill or elderly, nine times out of ten your relationship with the NHS is not a partnership. Some of the most vulnerable people in society who feel alienated are often those who have multiple and unmet health needs. Healthcare is not just curing all ill people

but making sure that people's whole lives are healthy. It is about removing those Berlin walls between health, social, and community services.

These words are particularly relevant to the prison population. Services therefore need to be seamless, characterised by co-operation and partnership between both clients and their support staff/carers. It is here that nurses can help by linking with local services and acting as advocates to ensure that their clients' needs are met. This is particularly important in areas where prisoners' lifestyles can be influenced and where attitudinal change can be brought about through, for example, the medium of health promotion and health education. The special relationship developed between nurse and prisoner provides an excellent vehicle for the provision of opportunistic health promotion in areas such as the re-education of eating habits and enhancement of a healthier approach to the individual's lifestyle in preparation for discharge.

Current situation

Currently prison nurses come from a range of backgrounds, each nurse bringing different skills and competences to the service, their common bond being their registration and the UKCC/NMC's Code of Professional Conduct (UKCC, 1992). There is no specific prison nurse qualification and the nurses who work in the service are qualified professional nurses. They have a qualification in one of the four branches of the profession with a range of experience and knowledge from a variety of different specialities. Many will have post-registration educational qualifications supported by their National Board for Nursing, Midwifery and Health Visiting. Others will have had specific training relevant to their area of practice but organised by academic or other professional bodies outside nursing such as National Vocational Qualifications (NVQs), degrees in law, psychology, etc. What is required is the development of a rather more specific professional identity for the nurse practising in prison healthcare. This would allow other healthcare colleagues to identify those elements of care that are specifically within the role and remit of the nurse in the prison healthcare environment. In 2002, the National Training Organisation (NTO) developed and published the custodial healthcare occupational standards for NVQ and SVQ. The standards will provide a baseline at NVQ level 3 of standards that all nursing staff will be required to demonstrate competence in. New entrant prison officers to prison healthcare will be required to undertake these qualifications. In addition there is a need for the nursing profession as a whole to understand the specialist contribution that nurses make within the prison environment and why their practice is so different. It is here that the new partnership arrangements with the NHS will be of value: the opportunity afforded for nurses outside prison healthcare to be exposed to the workings of prison life will do much to give others a better understanding of their role. In addition, staff will have the chance to attend multi-disciplinary and multi-agency educational sessions, designed to facilitate shared learning. This sort of shared learning will bring about a better understanding of individuals' different but nevertheless equally important contributions to the service.

Conflict between the duty to care and the duty to 'contain' prisoners will constantly challenge the role of the prison nurse. Willmott (1997) discusses this in her article on the dilemmas facing prison nurses in their day-to-day practice. However, this is not a view that is supported by the authors, who feel that although there will always be conflict and professional issues to address, it is possible to construct a healthcare environment within the shell of prison security. People vary in their presentation of everyday needs and prisoners are no exception. In order to provide responsive services to support prisoners it is essential that a wide range of knowledge, skills and experience is available to them through a multi-disciplinary team.

During the last two decades institutional models of care have been gradually replaced with a major change in philosophy and new services have developed based on primary healthcare and integrated services within the local community. The move to integrate prison healthcare with those services provided in the local NHS is timely and recognised in the joint NHS/Prison Service report:

> Prisoners are a transient population and most only spend a short time in custody before returning to the wider community taking with them their health and social problems. It makes sense therefore that time in prison should be used as an opportunity to ensure that prisoners receive the best health care possible.
>
> This has advantages for the individual, the community and the NHS. Good health care and health promotion in prisons should help enable individuals to function to their maximum potential on release, which may assist in reducing offending. It should also reduce morbidity in a high-risk section of the general population with medium and long-term reduction on the NHS.
>
> Better quality care together with improved links to the NHS are also likely to help prevent acute break down and consequent tragic incidents such as homicides or suicides by people with mental illness.
>
> (DOH, 1999)

Bringing about change

Changes in practice bring with them insecurity, fear and uncertainty, if not handled properly. If managed effectively, however, change can be stimulating and exciting, with the result that staff will lead improvement in service delivery. Strategies for change should be accompanied by the provision of a robust communication strategy and a staff educational package, designed to equip them with the new skills necessary to bring about and maintain requisite changes. A review and appraisal of the changes should take place a short period after their implementation. Along with any changes that are envisaged locally, there needs to be an educational exercise with members of the general public to remove some of the stereotyped opinions that so many of them hold about prisons and how they work. This is not an impossible task but it needs careful planning and good teamwork. Not all nurses can work within such constraints and there is no doubt that specific skills are required.

Conclusion

This chapter has looked at the multi-faceted role of the nurse in prison healthcare. This setting offers nurses a unique opportunity to be innovative and to develop a quality nursing service within a most challenging environment. It has emphasised the need to move away from a medically dominated service to a more flexible, patient-needs-led and multi-disciplinary team approach. This is advocated within the future strategy as outlined in *The Future Organisation of Prison Health Care* report (DOH, 1999). The development of an effective primary care service within prisons will mean doctors having to relinquish some aspects of team leadership to enable the delivery of a more flexible and patient sensitive service. These issues are currently being addressed as a result of the *Report of the Working Group on Doctors Working in Prisons* (DOH, 2001b). With the resultant new areas of responsibility, nurses and others will have to ensure that as their individual roles develop and change so do the ways they work and deploy their skills. These changes will have to be underpinned by current and ongoing research as well as a system of monitoring the quality and range of service provision. Successful multi-disciplinary teams are those where all professionals and team members are seen as equal and where the individuals within the team are recognised for their contribution, ability and skill base. Prison nurses along with colleagues are currently striving to provide a high quality, patient-centred service in often difficult surroundings and circumstances. Life in prison healthcare is challenging, stressful and frustrating, but it is an area of nursing that is ready for change and where there is the opportunity to use initiative and make a difference by enhancing the quality of care and life of clients/prisoners. The quality of care is now a key issue throughout the NHS. Nurses in prison healthcare are ideally placed to ensure that prisoners as patients receive the same level of care as they would receive in the NHS. However, for prison nurses to be effective within the prison healthcare service, they will need to be involved in influencing and structuring the political agenda that ultimately governs their practice environment. This means working together as a group professionally and effectively communicating with each other to share best practice, informed by the best available evidence (DOH, 2000). The biggest job of all is getting colleagues to understand and value the contribution that prison nurses can make to the future development of the prison healthcare service. This is a real challenge.

References

Alderman, C. (1999) Inside story. *Nursing Standard*, **13**(33), 14–16.

DOH (1999) *The Future Organisation of Prison Health Care*. Report by the Joint Prison Service and National Health Service Executive Working Group, Department of Health, London.

DOH (2000) *Nursing in Prisons*. Report by the Joint Prison Service and National Health Service Executive Working Group. Department of Health, London.

DOH (2001a) *Clinical Governance in Prison Health Care*. Department of Health/HM Prison Service, London.

DOH (2001b) *Report of the Working Group on Doctors Working in Prisons*. Department of Health, London.

Hancock, C. (1999) Partnership – the challenge for nursing. *Nursing Management*, **6**(3), 33–7.

Norman, A.E. & Parrish, A.A. (1999a) Prison nursing and the practice nurse model. *Practice Nursing*, **10**(1), 20–22.

Norman, A.E. & Parrish, A.A. (1999b) Prison healthcare: work environment and the nursing role. *British Journal of Nursing*, **8**(10), 653–6.

Richards, M.P.M. *et al.* (1995) *Imprisonment and Family Ties*. Home Office Research and Statistics Department, Research Bulletin No 38. HMSO, London.

NTO (2002) Custodial Healthcare Standards, NVQ and SVQ. National Training Organisation, London.

UKCC (1992) *Code of Professional Conduct for the Nurse, Midwife and Health Visitor*, 3rd edn. United Kingdom Central Council for Nursing, Midwifery and Health Visiting, London.

Willmott, Y. (1997) Prison nursing: the tension between custody and care. *British Journal of Nursing*, **6**(6), 333–6.

Further reading

RCN (1996a) *Issues in Nursing and Health – Women and Mental Health: The Nurse's Responsibilities*. Royal College of Nursing, London.

RCN (1996b) *Issues in Nursing and Health – Race, Ethnicity and Mental Health: The Nurse's Responsibilities*. Royal College of Nursing, London.

RCN (1996c) *Issues in Nursing and Health – Profiling Poverty: A Guide for Nurses in the Community*. Royal College of Nursing, London.

RCN (1997) *Issues in Nursing and Health – Ethical Dilemmas*. Royal College of Nursing, London.

RCN (1998) *Issues in Nursing and Health – Sexual Orientation and Mental Health: Guidance for Nurses*. Royal College of Nursing, London.

UKCC & University of Central Lancashire (1999) *Nursing in Secure Environments*. United Kingdom Central Council for Nursing, Midwifery and Health Visiting, London.

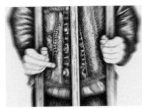

3 Prison Health
Policy Development

LINDSAY BATES AND LES STOREY

This chapter provides the reader with an essential overview of the prison health service, setting out the changes since the 1990s. The reader is encouraged to consider the past and the future as well as the present, and the chapter is designed to give a broader understanding of the political factors which have helped to shape current policy.

The development of healthcare and nursing in prisons is not something to which the prisons in England and Wales gave much attention before the late nineteenth century; not until 1902 was the first textbook on prison nursing published. The book you are now reading is the second book to be published in Britain on prison nursing and comes some 100 years after its predecessor, *Prison Hospital Nursing* by H. Smalley. This is not to suggest that there have not been considerable efforts to improve the conditions, healthcare and nursing services for prisoners in the intervening years.

Historical background

Until the late eighteenth century most offenders were punished by execution, corporal punishment, transportation or fine. Prisons were mostly used to house people before their trial or until their punishment was carried out, although financial crimes including debt have been punished by prison sentence since the fourteenth century. Prisons were also used to enforce the laws passed by the Church, the Universities at Oxford and Cambridge and the Stannery Courts of the tin mining districts in Devon and Cornwall.

Prisons had to be located in secure buildings and until the eighteenth century this often meant using space within existing buildings; usually part of the county town castle was employed as the county jail. During the eighteenth century new prisons became larger and in the 1770s the Corporation of Bath built a new prison in a similar style to that used in the large Georgian town houses being erected in Bath at the time.

John Howard (1726–90) was appointed as the High Sheriff of Bedfordshire in 1773. As sheriff he was responsible for the management of the county jail and commenced a period of extensive campaigning for changes in the management and organisation of prisons. He noted that the buildings were rarely purpose-built and usually in a poor state of repair; many prisons had no sewers or water supply; and urban prisons with cramped sites often had no exercise yards. Howard noted that disease and filth were brought into prisons by new inmates and recognised that 'many who went in healthy are in a few months changed to emaciated, dejected subjects'. John Howard systematically documented conditions in England's prisons and provided evidence to show why reforms were necessary. One of his first achievements was to obtain the Act of Parliament in 1774 that required separate rooms to be provided for sick prisoners and the appointment of an experienced surgeon or apothecary.

Infirmaries in early prisons were often in the governor's house but by the mid nineteenth century the main infirmary was usually in the administration block or adjacent to the male wings while the female one was located beside the female wing. At the end of the nineteenth century the size and scope of hospitals increased and new blocks that also contained reception facilities were built. Since the 1960s separate hospitals have been provided (English Heritage, 1999). In the late nineteenth century, the prison commissioners decided to organise a prison hospital staff for which candidates were required to pass through a probationary course of technical training, first aid and nursing. The first textbook on prison nursing, published in 1902 by His Majesty's Stationery Office, was described as a manual of first aid and nursing for the prison hospital staff. *Prison Hospital Nursing* was written by Herbert Smalley MD, Medical Inspector of Prisons (Smalley, 1902). This book was aimed at the prison hospital officer as it was not until much later (in the 1980s) that qualified nurses were actively encouraged to join the prison health services as healthcare officers.

Dr Smalley's book reflects many of the attitudes of the time among doctors and nursing staff, and many nurses today would be insulted by the tone of his writing. However, if one can overcome this there are some important messages that are as important today as they were then. In particular, he says:

Disabuse your mind of the idea that the prison is a den of iniquity, the warder a surly guardian and that because you have only criminals to deal with they do not require the same skill, care and attention when ill as is deemed requisite for those more happily situated. Enough for you to remember that they're probably more frail morally and perhaps also mentally and physically than those met with outside the prison wall yet they are as capable of being influenced by care, gentleness and upright conduct as most other human beings. Who can tell what good may be done by a kind action and good example when a stubborn nature is softened by the levelling hand of illness.

Dr Smalley gives advice and guidance to nurses to care for their own health, to eat well, have exercise and open air and to maintain personal hygiene. Less helpful is his reminder to nurses that they are not doctors, must pay strict obedience and fidelity to his orders and never express an adverse criticism upon the course of treatment being pursued. These sentiments would not be acceptable to nurses in the twenty-first century. Perhaps most interesting is the fact that Dr Smalley identifies many of the same issues that were found in the UKCC *Nursing in Secure Environments* study in 1999 (UKCC & University of Central Lancashire, 1999). In particular, he notes that the range of health needs of prisoners is extremely diverse and includes severe mental illness, personality disorder, poor physical health and trauma. The UKCC study also noted the effects of drug and alcohol dependency on the prison population and the need for effective primary care and health promotion.

Background – policy development

In 1996 Her Majesty's Inspectorate of Prisons for England and Wales issued a discussion paper *Patient or Prisoner* (HMIP, 1996a) posing the question 'Are people in prison with health problems prisoners first or patients and how best might their health needs be met?' The favoured option within the paper was that healthcare for prisoners should be provided by the NHS. In response to the paper, a joint working party was established between HM Prison Service and the NHS Executive to:

- address the issues in *Patient or Prisoner* (HMIP, 1996a) and other relevant documents
- develop practical proposals for change that would:
    - deliver care for prisoners equivalent to that of the general population
    - take account of the wider prison and NHS agendas
    - take account of the views of key stakeholders.

The report of the working party, *The Future Organisation of Prison Health Care* (DOH, 1999b) was published in March 1999. This report endorsed the existing aim for prison healthcare to 'give prisoners access to the same quality and range of health care services as the general public receives from the National Health Service'. It identified considerable variation in the organisation, delivery, quality, funding and effectiveness of prison healthcare and its links with the NHS. No two prisons can be regarded as the same, largely because of historic legacy, *ad hoc* development and the relative isolation from the NHS. Prison healthcare has often been reactive rather than proactive, over-medicalised and health needs assessments the exception rather than the rule. Healthcare provision has suffered from a lack of direction, poor lines of communication and confused accountability. The arrangements for the continuing professional development of healthcare staff have not been well established and there have not been effective ways to monitor the outcomes of care.

As a consequence of the recommendations of the report of the working party (DOH, 1999b) a formal partnership between the prison service and the NHS has been established. Two new units came into existence in spring 2000, the Prison Health Policy Unit and the Prison Health Task Force.

The Prison Health Policy Unit that replaced the prison service Directorate of Health Care is responsible for the development of prison health policy, drawing on and integrating with the wider NHS policies. The Policy Unit advises the Prisons Board, the NHS Executive and ministers on prison health policy with the Head of the Unit, a member of the Prison Service Executive Board. The Prison Health Task Force was established to help support prisons and health authorities to drive forward the assessment of prisoners' health needs and the changes identified by the prison health improvement programmes. The Task Force will be established for three to five years to act as a change agent and facilitator to achieve the objectives outlined in *The Future Organisation of Prison Health Care* report (DOH, 1999b).

This report identified the significant role played by nurses in the delivery of health services for prisoners. It noted: 'Prisons where nurses had been empowered as organisational managers and clinical leaders appeared to have more consistent and professional delivery of care.' However, the opportunity to use more nurses cost-effectively has in many instances been missed owing to inflexible employment practices and inexperience of managing nursing terms and conditions of employment. Some nursing staff commented that they were often required to perform tasks inappropriate to their skills resulting in less than optimum use of their abilities. The report also noted that the morale of both nursing medical staff and healthcare officers appeared low and that confusion around the management of healthcare within prisons was illustrated by the variety of job titles and backgrounds of those undertaking management roles. The working party report also examined the roles of nursing and healthcare officers within the multi-disciplinary team. Given the variation in size and type of prison establishments, the report could not be precise about the model of nursing services. However, nursing leadership was recognised as requiring support by governors and other managers; in particular, nurses must be enabled to practise within their ethical framework, the Code of Professional Conduct (UKCC, 1992). The working party concluded that the roles of nurses in prisons should be based on flexible and effective models of nursing competences. Nursing care and healthcare centres should be led by qualified nurses who should have ready access to the governor's senior management team and models of clinical supervision for nurses should be introduced. The working party reported shortly before publication of the 1999 Department of Health strategy document for nursing *Making a Difference* (DOH, 1999a). This strategy document identified that nurses, midwives and health visitors are vital to the NHS and to the nation, making a real difference to people's lives. People trust nurses and have confidence in them. It also identified that the context of care is changing and that nurses, midwives and health visitors face new challenges that are often constrained by structures that limit development and innovation. *Making a Difference* (DOH, 1999a) set a number of challenges to strengthen the nursing, midwifery and health visiting contribution to health and healthcare. These two reports created a context and background for change in prison nursing that had not been available before.

While policy changes were taking place in England and Wales, the strategy and policy direction for nurses working in Northern Ireland and Scotland had advanced separately and in many instances significantly ahead of policy and strategy development for prison nurses in England and Wales.

In addition to these government-led initiatives, the United Kingdom Central Council for Nursing, Midwifery and Health Visiting published the results of a UK-wide study, *Nursing in Secure Environments* (UKCC & University of Central Lancashire, 1999). This project was a scoping study into the issues involved in the work of practitioners working in secure environments. The need for this project had arisen from a number of concerns that the UKCC had, including the rising number of calls and correspondence to the Council's professional advisory service stimulated by the ongoing national enquiries into services in mental health and prison services. The scoping study was the first time the Council had comprehensively analysed the issues facing practitioners who work in secure environments. A total of 440 nurses working in prison health services in the UK, 338 of them from England and Wales, provided data and input to the UKCC project, which provides an excellent source of information about the challenges of providing healthcare to the prison population and highlights a number of significant challenges for prison healthcare staff. It particularly notes the challenge of the competing cultures and the tensions between therapy and security. The UKCC report cites a quote by a healthcare co-ordinator in Day (1983):

> The clients with whom we deal are complex individuals, some are manipulators and/or malingerers, some are genuine, some are drug addicts and many have alcohol problems. Some use the system, others utilise it. They are men, women and trans-sexuals. Some are retarded, some psychotic, some depressed, some normal and they present a variety of physical conditions including diabetes, heart problems, multiple sclerosis, arthritis and even pregnancy. On the whole the nurse/patient relationship is congenial but this does not alter the fact that these individuals lead a life much different from our own and have a value system that may not correspond to ours.

Shortly after the publication of the *Nursing in Secure Environments* study (UKCC & University of Lancashire, 1999), and in response to increasing concerns about the problems in prison healthcare and nursing, the Prisons Minister, Paul Boateng MP, and the Health Minister, Lord Hunt, established a working party to consider the development of prison nursing with particular reference to healthcare officers. The working party objectives were:

(1)   To consider the future prison nursing workforce with particular reference to healthcare officers to identify approaches to be taken to ensure an integrated nursing workforce best placed to meet the health needs of prisoners.
(2)   To identify the actions needed to meet the healthcare needs of prisoners and have the potential to make rapid improvements to the division of healthcare.

The working party reported in October 2000 and made a total of 34 recommendations to achieve the overall objectives of the working party and to develop a nursing workforce able to meet the health needs of prisoners for the future. The Prison Health Policy Unit and Task Force were charged with taking forward these recommendations to enhance the services provided within prison healthcare.

The prison population and assessed health needs

The daily prison population in 2000 was approximately 65 000 and was predicted to rise to 72 000 by 2002 (as of May 2002 the prison population stood at approximately 70 000). During the period April 1998–99 staff providing healthcare in prisons in England and Wales handled over two million consultations with inmates. About two-thirds of these involved contact with a nurse or a healthcare officer. The population is predominantly a male population who drink and smoke heavily, have more active health problems than the population at large and show evidence of adverse health effects on their lifestyle. Prisoners suffer from high levels of mental disorder, drug abuse and general poor health (Birmingham *et al.*, 1996; Mason *et al.*, 1997).

The Office for National Statistics *Study into Psychiatric Morbidity amongst Prisoners* (ONS, 1998) identified a large number of prisoners with mental health disorders. A high proportion of respondents presented with significant neurotic symptoms (anxiety, depression and phobias) ranging from 39% of male sentenced prisoners to 75% of female remand prisoners. Rates for all groups are much higher than similar household surveys (men 12%, women 18%). Psychosis, substance misuse, paranoid and borderline personality disorders were the most common types of disorder. Men were much more likely to report alcohol abuse and dependence on drugs in the year before coming into prison.

The prison health workforce

Pegram (in an unpublished 1997 dissertation from the University of Bradford) records that, towards the end of the nineteenth century, the Gladstone Report of 1895 argued that the prison system should be more flexible and discriminating, capable both of responding to the needs of individual prisoners and also of helping to make prisoners better men and women when they left the prison. As the different needs of prisoners were recognised so specialists from outside were introduced into prisons, the earliest of these in the nineteenth century being the doctor, who was assisted by prison officers called hospital officers – more recently named healthcare officers.

Within the United Kingdom there are three prison services: England and Wales; Scotland; and Northern Ireland. These have developed to reflect the needs of populations and at a different pace albeit in much the same direction. In 1992 the prison service for England and Wales set targets to increase the proportion of registered nurses in its workforce to 75% of the non-medical workforce by the year 2000 (Wool, 1992). By March 1999 this stood at 70.6% although the composition of the registered nurse workforce was not always best suited to the health needs of the prisoners but more to the availability of nursing applicants.

Since the early 1900s the prison service has been largely dependent on prison officers who were trained in the delivery of healthcare for prisoners. Prison officers in the latter part of the twentieth century undertook training of six months' duration to equip them for working in prison healthcare. The curriculum included aspects of physical and mental healthcare that would enable them to meet the requirements of the Health Care Standing Order 13 (HMIP, 1996b):

- carrying out basic nursing care and such specialist nursing care within their competence
- observing patients in their charge and alerting the medical officer to any matters relating to the health or treatment of a patient which are considered to warrant medical attention
- keeping accurate records of medicine administered and other significant nursing duties undertaken as required by the managing medical officer
- advising medical officers on the statutory provisions, standing orders and Headquarters instructions and general guidance relevant to the performance of their duties generally of the procedure in a particular case.

In 1992 the Director of Healthcare Services for Prisoners, Dr Rosemary Wool, issued a policy statement saying:

> The experience, skills and interests of individual members of the nursing staff make it necessary for management to determine the appropriate skill mix with advice from the Directorate of Health Care. The role of nursing staff will be extended and enhanced to include services such as counselling and health education. The greater emphasis in future will be on preventative medicine, health education and health promotion which can be expected to evolve from the establishment of the Health Care Services for Prisoners and will provide further opportunities for research work making the job of nursing staff more satisfying and rewarding. There are advantages in nursing grades gravitating between the National Health Service and the Nursing Service for prisoners. It is one viable means of refreshing prison nursing and keeping the service in tune with the ethos and methods of the National Health Service.
>
> (Wool, 1992)

The Future Organisation of Prison Health Care report (DOH, 1999b) noted that 'Over the last few years registered nurses have been recruited but without a meaningful assessment of the knowledge and skills required. Their particular competences have not often been utilised to the full.' The report contained an aspiration that in future all nursing care would be under the supervision of a first level registered nurse. It also sought to move towards the separating of custodial and nursing functions and suggested that this might have an impact on healthcare officers. It stated that healthcare officers who satisfied selection criteria should be enabled to undertake nurse training in the light of assessed health needs and skills shortages. Those unable to acquire nursing qualifications would undertake appropriate therapeutic roles in the context of developed regimes for dealing with prisoners with mental disorders and, within a multi-disciplinary healthcare team, healthcare officers would continue to play a key role. This lack of clarity about the future role of healthcare officers was one of the key issues to be addressed by the 1999 working party to consider the development of prison nursing. The report produced by the working party *Nursing in Prisons* (DOH, 2000a) provides a strategy for the development of nursing care delivery for the beginning of the twenty-first century.

Strategies for prison nursing

Healthcare teams

The working party established by ministers to consider the development of prison nursing brought together representatives from the prison service healthcare teams. This included doctors, nurses and healthcare officers, senior managers, policy makers and significantly, the two key unions – the Royal College of Nursing and the Prison Officers' Association – and the UKCC.

The working party recognised the importance of making the best use of the skills available in the service and likely to be available in the future. It identified the need to reflect the wider healthcare service trends in the NHS and the flexible use of staff. It also suggested the development of national occupational standards and the introduction of modular competence-based training linked to assessed patient need. Clinical governance and work patterns were other issues needing further consideration.

Furthermore, the working party identified the special nature of the prison setting, the range of prison populations and the high rate of prisoner movement between prisons. The moratorium on the recruitment of healthcare officers had been lifted in December 1999, and the working party confirmed that prison healthcare should be delivered by healthcare teams with a range of qualifications and competences linked to the health needs of prisoners as reflected in the wider NHS. In particular the report recognised the nursing team as including all staff engaged in nursing care, that is, nurses and healthcare officers and nursing assistants. The wider healthcare team includes doctors, pharmacists and therapists working in prison healthcare.

Education and training

The prison nursing strategy outlined in the *Nursing in Prisons* report (DOH, 2000a) was underpinned by a competence-based approach to training, performance management, recruitment and selection. It sought to develop an integrated approach to nursing in prisons, engaging healthcare officers and nurses employed by the prison service as well as nurses working in the NHS or alternative employers and providing services to prisoners.

This competence-based approach was one of the key recommendations of the *Nursing in Secure Environments* study (UKCC & University of Central Lancashire, 1999) and reflected the need for nurses and healthcare officers to have skills in mental health, general nursing and the custodial environment including some aspects of security. This was indeed the premise of Dr Smalley's textbook in 1902 although not expressed in the same way (Smalley, 1902). The challenge in this approach was to develop a framework of training that would be acceptable to nurses and healthcare officers and that would prepare them for working in prison healthcare. Modern nurse training and discipline officer training would provide some of the skills and competences required but no single route of training would encompass the full range of competences required.

The competence-based approach can be translated into a national vocational qualification (NVQ) which assesses the competence of an individual to undertake the tasks required within a given area of employment. The prison service has for a number of years been committed to developing the NVQ approach for its discipline staff and this approach was considered by the working party to be the most appropriate one to develop and articulate the skills for nursing in prisons. Nurses, however, have not been very enthusiastic about NVQs and have sought qualifications that were validated by the academic institutions or the nursing educational boards. In recognition of this, the working party recommended that the NVQ in custodial healthcare should be developed in a way that enabled nurses to achieve academic credits for further study at diploma or degree level.

The Custodial Health Care National Training Organisation commissioned work to develop the functional map and competence framework for nursing staff working in custodial settings. In recognition of the need to develop more creative career paths and break down some of the institutional barriers, the custodial healthcare qualification will be applicable to staff working outside prisons and other custodial or secure care settings.

The nature of nurse education in the UK was scrutinised by the UKCC Commission for Education in 1999. The final report *Fitness for Practice* (UKCC, 1999) made a number of recommendations including provision of the opportunity for individuals with relevant experience to gain exemption from part of the common foundation programme for nurse registration. This would, within the new proposals, reduce some of the frustration felt by healthcare officers who could not previously have their experience recognised and who would have had to undertake the full three-year programme. The future strategy for nursing, therefore, will seek to meet the requirements for credits towards the common foundation programme for nurses.

Conversely, the custodial training that nurses undertake will gain credits towards discipline officer training for those who wish to pursue a role as prison officer in the future. This more flexible and integrated approach to training has at the time of writing still to be tried and tested but has gained support and encouragement from all key parties and was fully endorsed by ministers.

Following the publication of *The Future Organisation of Prison Health Care* (DOH, 1999b) in March 1999, the partnership between the NHS and the prison service was to be underpinned by an assessment of the health needs of prisoners in each establishment. This has led to the essential redesigning and reshaping of healthcare in prisons and the new responsibility for local health authorities to include the health needs of the local prison population in its planning and resource allocation.

Models for developing skills and competence of healthcare staff may then be based upon these health needs assessments; similarly, the occupational standards required for the healthcare team to deliver an appropriate service may be identified so that training may be provided for members of the healthcare team. These occupational standards will contribute to the occupational standards that will form the basis of the custodial healthcare NVQ. The core occupational standards in prison healthcare can be identified as:

- safety and security
- assessment and observation including risk assessment, risk management to reduce self-harm, management of violence and aggression, therapies and treatment including cognitive behaviour therapy and psychosocial interventions, knowledge of offending behaviour and appropriate legislation, and report-writing

- jail craft (*sic*) – a term used to describe the prison context and culture
- practical nursing skills, first aid, administration and management of medications.

(based on UKCC & University of Central Lancashire, 1999)

A hierarchy of competences was described by the working party ranging from *cannot do satisfactorily* (Level 1), through to *expert practitioner* at Level 6. It was agreed that all staff working in prison nursing should be able to perform the full range of competences satisfactorily, without assistance and/or constant supervision.

New staff entering prison healthcare would undergo an induction programme based on these competences, which should commence in the first month of appointment at basic level to ensure staff were adequately prepared for working within the prison healthcare setting. They would be expected to achieve competence in a number of mandatory occupational standards within one year of commencement. This clear policy statement was the first time that the induction and further training requirements of staff working in prison healthcare were identified. The significance of this approach was endorsed by the professional body, staff organisations and ministers, and supported by additional funding for a three-year period to enable the training to become embedded within the prison service.

Career progression

Nursing careers at the end of the twentieth and beginning of the twenty-first centuries are extremely diverse and provide enormous opportunities for nurses working in a variety of settings. A career that includes experience of working with prisoners can be rich and rewarding; however, much as the experience for nurses working in prisons should be seen as career-enhancing, this has not always been the case, and prior to the *Nursing in Prisons* report (DOH, 2000a) nurses working in prisons felt unrecognised and undervalued. *Nursing in Prisons* sought to develop flexible career paths for nurses and healthcare officers with career progression based on the identified needs of the service, and the individual's assessed competence and ability to take on more complex, more specialist service roles or management roles.

The importance of training, experience and performance being nationally accredited was to demonstrate its relevance not only to the prison setting but also to other settings outside the prison service. Many nurses move in and out of prison healthcare owing to the wide variety of job opportunities. Occupational standards-based training and experience in the prison healthcare service is more likely to be seen as career enhancement, especially when supported with recognition through academic credits. This will attract more nurses to the service, aid their recruitment and retention and support career progression in prison healthcare management and other areas of the prison service. Healthcare officers also continue to be important members of the healthcare team, representing a substantial pool of skills and a unique understanding of the prison setting and the prison population. The occupational standards and competence base should ensure that healthcare officers as well as nurses are equipped to meet the needs of prisoners. Healthcare officers are now expected to comply with the NMC codes of conduct and training requirements.

Terms and conditions of service

The terms and conditions of work for healthcare officers and nurses have differed and created a source of tension and frustration for staff and managers alike. For instance, nursing staff employed under Whitley Council terms and conditions work shorter hours than healthcare officers and they are able to work and be paid for overtime. Healthcare officers are not paid overtime but have a time off in lieu system. In addition to the result of staff becoming overtired, which in itself contributes to the cycle of sickness, absence and low morale, the fact that staff are engaged under different terms and conditions of service also works against harmony and integration within the nursing team. Furthermore, problems in recruitment and retention of nurses have had an impact. While most prison officers join the prison service as their chosen career and those choosing to work in healthcare tend to stay for many years, nurses choose to join a profession that may take them into many areas, including prisons. As working in prison may form only a part of nurses' careers, they may be perceived as not having the same level of commitment as prison officers. These tensions require skilled management and team-building and could be seen as an opportunity to develop a dynamic workforce that is re-appraising its skills base to meet the needs of the population in a creative way.

The prison service has not historically made use of flexible approaches to staff employment, such as the use of part-time staff or short-term contracts to deal with variations in activity. However, changes are rapidly taking place within the prison service causing it to become more flexible and thereby attract staff from a wide range of backgrounds and communities. Further initiatives to attract and retain staff from black and ethnic minority communities that may better reflect the diversity of the prison population are also beginning to emerge.

Nurses and healthcare officers who work within prison healthcare will continue to have training and development needs beyond their initial induction and competences. The NMC (UKCC, 1996, 1998) requires nurses to demonstrate the equivalent of five days' worth of study activity relevant to their area of clinical practice every three years as a pre-requisite for registration (post-registration education and practice – PREP) and continuing professional development (CPD) requirements. This requirement has now been embraced by the prison service for all staff and will be reflected in work plans and staff training requirements in the future. Registered nurses are required by the NMC to maintain and update a nursing portfolio. In 2000 the prison service developed its own portfolio for all nursing staff, including non-registered healthcare staff.

Other initiatives within the wider health services have identified training requirements to which nurses working in prisons should have access; for example, the *Mental Health National Service Framework* (DOH, 2000b) identified the need to develop the workforce in new and imaginative ways. These requirements will have an impact on staff working with prisoners as much as on those working with the wider community managing the healthcare team, and nurses within prison healthcare will have the same need for further education as their colleagues in the team.

Nursing leadership

The leadership and management of such a diverse group of staff to meet the varied needs of prisoners provides a further challenge. *The Future Organisation of Prison Health Care* (DOH, 1999b) recommended that managers of prison healthcare should be competent as managers *per se* and form part of the senior management team in the prison. Healthcare manager posts should be open to anybody with development skills and competences in managing healthcare, and their post-basic nurse education and training should build on their individual needs and the competences required within the prison setting.

The need to develop effective nurse leaders was identified in *Making a Difference*, the Department of Health's strategy for nursing (DOH, 1999a). In the strategy it recognises that the programme of modernisation within the NHS presents a challenging leadership agenda:

> We need visionary leadership to help build modern, dependable services and to inspire and sustain the commitment of nurses, midwives and health visitors during a period of significant change. Strong nursing, midwifery and health visiting leadership is needed at every level.

This is also the case within the prison service, particularly with the development of inter-agency and multi-disciplinary team working, and the needs to improve quality and practice through clinical governance and provide effective management of clinical services and corporate functions.

Making a Difference (DOH, 1999a) suggests that organisations should have a clear understanding of where weaknesses in leadership capacity and capability present a risk to clinical standards. The best organisations will have identified measures to close the gap. NHS organisations were expected to:

- review their current provision and investment in clinical leadership development to ensure nurses, midwives and health visitors have access to appropriate opportunities
- ensure that all nurses, midwives and health visitors can benefit from a robust system of review and personal development planning
- invest in continuing professional development to support clinical governance and in the development and support of clinical leaders
- use clinical supervision and statutory midwifery supervision to help identify, support and develop nurse, midwife and health visitor leaders and potential leaders
- establish effective succession planning and support and coach nurses, midwives and health visitors who aspire to leadership positions by providing opportunities for informal development such as mentoring, shadowing, job swaps, secondments and participation in learning sets
- ensure that nurses, midwives and health visitors from black and ethnic minority groups and part-time staff, who have traditionally been under-represented in career development activity, have equality of opportunity.

These criteria apply within the prison service. *The Future Organisation of Prison Health Care* (DOH, 1999b) recommended that nursing should be under the direction of a registered nurse; this in itself poses challenges where the registered nurse may not be the head of healthcare. This is further compounded by the requirements for clinical governance: it is the governor who is responsible for management and quality of prison healthcare and it is his or her duty to see that prisoners receive good healthcare.

However, the governor is expected not to provide direct management and leadership but to ensure that healthcare is effectively managed. Nurses have made a significant contribution to corporate and strategic management, and this needs to continue. Opportunities to develop generic management skills and to enter corporate and strategic roles must be maintained to ensure that decision-making is properly informed by nursing knowledge. It may be easier therefore to separate the issues of management of healthcare and governance of healthcare, and the healthcare manager should be directly responsible to the governor for the quality of healthcare being delivered by the healthcare team. The healthcare manager needs to be part of the senior management team of the prison, and should have in place ways of organising healthcare services that:

- enable the governor, who is not expected to have clinical expertise or in-depth knowledge of health issues, to have assurance of the quality of healthcare that is being delivered in the prison for which he or she is responsible
- enable the healthcare team to deliver acceptable healthcare and recruit and retain staff to enable these standards to be met
- provide monthly reports to the governor on all aspects relating to clinical governance
- ensure that individual members of the healthcare team work to agreed clinical and professional standards
- give members of prison healthcare staff, prisoners and families access to independent advice if they feel there are healthcare problems that have not been resolved internally.

For nursing leadership, this means nursing should be led by a suitably qualified and competent registered nurse to ensure appropriate supervision and quality standards. This does *not* mean that nurses must carry out all duties. It *does* mean that nurses leading nursing within prisons should be equipped with the appropriate leadership qualities and skills. Poor clinical leadership leads to poor standards of care. This is unacceptable and will be highlighted more readily by the new arrangements for clinical governance (DOH, 1999a). Clinical leadership programmes, such as the scheme run by the RCN and the LEO (leading empowered organisations) programme run by the National Leadership Centre, have shown how development programmes for clinical leaders involving action learning can have very positive results. Similar work to develop staff involvement and leadership is ongoing across a number of NHS organisations. Programmes such as these need to become the norm rather than the exception. *Nursing in Prisons* (DOH, 2000a) recommended the introduction of a management development programme for healthcare managers. This initiative will build on the recommendations from *Making a Difference* (DOH, 1999a) and *The Future Organisation of Prison Health Care* (DOH, 1999b) to provide leaders who can take the service and the nursing workforce forward. In line with the NHS, the prison service needs nurse leaders who can establish direction and purpose; inspire, motivate and empower teams around common goals;

and produce real improvements in clinical practice, quality and services. Leaders are needed who are motivated, self-aware, socially skilled and able to work together with others across professional and organisational boundaries. Aspiring leaders need to be identified, supported and developed. Senior colleagues have an obligation to spot and nurture talent, to encourage and develop leadership qualities and skills and to create a professional and organisational climate that enables the next generation of leaders to challenge orthodoxy, to take risks and to learn from experience (DOH, 1999b).

Challenges for nurses in prisons

Much is made of the custody versus care roles in prison healthcare. This is no longer an acceptable line of discussion. Nurses and healthcare staff have to recognise that they are providing care in a custodial setting and that they have to integrate their responsibilities. Not to do so would be to deny prisoners the optimum healthcare that they have a right to expect and receive. This clearly is not a simple task, and requires professional and personal maturity and confidence. The prison system will always have security as its priority for staff, prisoners and visitors. This is also the way the service is able to maintain the confidence of the public and government. This does not mean, however, that the health and well-being of prisoners is not also uppermost in the service's concerns. The clear link between mental health, alcohol and drug abuse, and crime demonstrates the potential for healthcare to have a positive impact on re-offending and the running of a prison.

The prison services in the UK are going through a significant period of change and challenge that provides an opportunity to enhance the quality and diversity of care provided to prisoners to meet their assessed needs. Equipping nurses with the appropriate competences, support and leadership will enable us to meet these challenges and take prison healthcare into the twenty-first century with innovative and imaginative nurses providing high quality care.

References

Birmingham, L., Mason, D. & Grubin, D. (1996) Prevalence of mental disorder in remand prisoners: consecutive case study. *British Medical Journal*, **313**, 1521–4.

Day, C. (1983) The challenge: health vs security. *The Canadian Nurse*, **79**(7), 34–6.

DOH (1999a) *Making a Difference*. Department of Health, London.

DOH (1999b) *The Future Organisation of Prison Health Care*. Report by the Joint Prison Service and National Health Service Executive Working Group. Department of Health, London.

DOH (2000a) *Nursing in Prisons*. Report by the Joint Prison Service and National Health Service Executive Working Group. Department of Health, London.

DOH (2000b) *The Mental Health National Service Framework*. The Stationery Office, London.

English Heritage (1999) *Behind Bars – The Hidden Architecture of England's Prisons*. English Heritage, London.

HMIP (1996a) *Patient or Prisoner? A New Strategy for Health Care in Prisons*. Discussion paper. HM Inspectorate of Prisons, London.

HMIP (1996b) *Health Care Standing Order 13*. HM Prison Service, London.

Mason, D., Birmingham, L. & Grubin, D. (1997) Substance misuse in remand prisoners: a consecutive case study. *British Medical Journal*, **315**, 667–73.

ONS (1998) *Study into Psychiatric Morbidity amongst Prisoners*. Office for National Statistics, London.

Smalley, H. (1902) *Prison Hospital Nursing*. HMSO, London.

UKCC (1992) *Code of Professional Conduct for the Nurse, Midwife and Health Visitor*. 3rd edn. United Kingdom Central Council for Nursing, Midwifery and Health Visiting, London.

UKCC (1996) *Guidelines for Professional Practice*. United Kingdom Central Council for Nursing, Midwifery and Health Visiting, London.

UKCC (1998) *PREP and You*. United Kingdom Central Council for Nursing, Midwifery and Health Visiting, London.

UKCC (1999) *Fitness for Practice*. United Kingdom Central Council for Nursing, Midwifery and Health Visiting, London.

UKCC & University of Central Lancashire (1999) *Nursing in Secure Environments*. United Kingdom Central Council for Nursing, Midwifery and Health Visiting, London.

Wool, R. (1992) *Nursing Service for Prisoners: Policy Statement*. Directorate of Health Care, London.

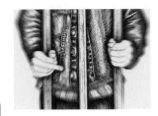

4 Understanding and Changing the Dynamics of the Prison Culture

SALLY THOMSON AND ALAN A. PARRISH

The prison culture is complex and is influenced by historical attitudes. The combined attitudes of the public, of prison staff and of prisoners create unique challenges for the prison nurse. There are common cultural themes in all prison establishments, and some unique cultural differences between prisons. This chapter will help the reader to understand prison culture; in doing so, it may suggest opportunities for positive changes.

Introduction

This chapter explores the elements of behaviour that make up the culture and dynamics of group behaviour. The culture of a prison is unique, and different from any other work environment in which a nurse might practise. Nursing and our modern philosophies in health and caring are new to prison healthcare, and both nurses and the prison healthcare team have to learn different ways of working. Trying to achieve change in such an atmosphere is difficult and can be frustrating.

Understanding change processes and applying different perspectives explored in this chapter will help the reader to understand better what is going on, to consider ways around problems and to make a difference.

People do not act only as individuals: we are all influenced by the people we mix with, both in our social and domestic life and when we are in the work situation (Hayes & Orrell, 1993). In everyday situations we behave in ways that fit the particular context we are in, and every dynamic situation that we are in has its own set of expectations about the proper way to behave; fitting in with these is important if we are to be accepted by the group. In prison life, this can be very difficult for a nurse, who has to work within a code of practice set by the UKCC (UKCC, 1992); some work colleagues do not always understand this. Some nurses may have been subject to peer pressure for so long that they are unaware of how far they have moved from caring practice and philosophies.

There are sanctions within any group for putting pressure on individuals to behave in a way that conforms to the norm of the group. These sanctions can vary from innuendoes – which are difficult to identify – or a mild rebuke from colleagues, to the extremes of bullying or total isolation. They can be formal in terms of a disciplinary procedure, or informal as peer group pressure. Often the informal sanctions are the most difficult for an individual to handle. It is the nature of most humans to wish to belong to social groups; therefore sanctions are particularly painful and may make us change behaviour to achieve a sense of belonging. Unknowingly, we sabotage standards of care that we value when this happens.

Culture

A culture has been defined as a 'system of meanings and cultures', shared by an identifiable group (Malim & Birch, 1998). To assess our work environment accurately, it is important to consider the influence of the culture that has developed and the reasons for the direction it has taken. Pennington (1986) stresses the importance of the social context as having a major influence upon individuals and their behaviour. Within a prison culture, sub-cultures may develop that offer individuals different sub-groups; each may provide values, attitudes, laws and moral codes of conduct, and influence the individual's self-esteem and positive or negative self-perception. The culture is crucial to the way we are socialised into work, and may be something that should be considered when orienting new or agency staff into the social environment of a prison with its unique, enclosed and discipline-dominated way of life.

In particular, the interface between the work of prison officers and that of nurses needs to be overtly addressed, examining both complementary and differing modes of practice. It may be worth looking at the marked contrasts between containment/discipline and caring. (These are areas that do cause concern and conflict for nurses.) For example, consider the opportunities that are afforded in areas of care with less restricted environments than those found in prisons. A nurse could spend time with a patient perceived as needing some 'quality time' in a flexible service in a manner that would be totally impossible within a prison healthcare service. Or again, consoling a patient who is grieving or upset over a particular incident is relatively easy in many more conventional healthcare situations, but this may be not so easy in a prison setting. This is a challenge for a nurse, who has to be innovative and use initiative to work within the restrictive regimes of a prison while still producing a high level of care and making the atmosphere as therapeutic as possible.

Looking at this situation from a prison officer's perspective, unless time is spent explaining nursing actions and rationale, it may look as if the nurse is set on sabotaging prison routines and regimes. This is an area where good communication and understanding of each other's roles is essential if a patient-centred service is to be established. Agreed care plans may bridge this divide. Or a nurse may set up a case conference or team meeting to bring these contrasts to the fore and to look for acceptable compromises, while still valuing the perspective of an opposing ideology; this will take some sensitive communication on the nurse's part. Or again, offering each other clinical supervision may be a useful area to address.

Sub-groups

Sub-groups exist within team cultures: a group with a shared interest in sport or music, a social set, or a group of deviants who exert pressure on others and impede progress, etc. Comparing group behaviours makes it obvious that each group has a different ethos, set of standards and purpose. An individual's behaviour and use of language within one group may be compared to the individual's behaviour and use of language when in the midst of a different group of people. It is also an interesting exercise to look at the contrasting views of groups, for example, attitudes to work, people, ethical issues and particularly other groups.

Group members who have formed a social set are easy to work with as a group, since their relationship skills are such that issues are resolved in an adult manner; their goodwill can be built upon, and their enthusiasm can be maximised. The deviants are different and may be harder to relate to; they could cause the nurse to feel de-skilled and apprehensive.

Culture and control

There is little doubt that a prison has a unique culture and a nurse has to understand the rules and workings of it and the key players within it to function successfully. Being in this environment for the first time may be difficult and the nurse may need a period of conscious adjustment where the reflective processes (described elsewhere in this book) could be usefully maximised. To make this transition, support from a mentor, preceptor or clinical supervisor could be helpful.

Society at large expects to be protected from members who, for whatever reason, are deemed by the courts to be worthy of detention at Her Majesty's pleasure for a period of time depending on the severity of their individual crimes. Punishment is seen to be the prison sentence and the individual's exclusion from life in the community. While staff cannot be expected to expunge from their minds a person's previous history and behaviour, this must be put to one side when dealing with the individual. There is a body of evidence that shows that people behave according to others' expectations: if, for example, people are treated as inferior they will respond in a way that reinforces that perception. If people are valued, this is evident in healthy adult therapeutic or professional relationships that lead to atmospheres where tensions are minimised and acceptable codes of behaviour are normal (Coon, 1998). There is always the danger of staff taking a high-handed approach to prisoners and missing the chance of using an occasion to set an example from which the prisoner may learn. Although control is one of the central features of the prison culture and is an integral and important facet of the regimes in prison life, it is nevertheless a fact of life that a prison can only be run effectively and efficiently with the co-operation of the prisoners.

What happens to people after their conviction is clearly a matter of importance to society generally. It is not only the offenders who are affected. Crime is a burden on society, which suffers in many ways, not just in measurable cost-outcomes. All institutions face the dangers of being closed environments. The dangers and consequences of this happening are reflected in the many inquiry reports on hospitals in the past decade (DOH, 1992). While there is much to be done to get prison life right and to expose the current staff to the changes that are envisaged for the future, the truth is that we have outgrown the vindictiveness of the Victorian attitude towards prisoners. However, prisoners are not always given the respect that they should have as individuals – staff sometimes forget that the punishment is the prisoner's sentence. (Everyone has the right to dignity and respect.)

There is, therefore, still much work to be done in respect of changing the attitude of society to the rehabilitation of offenders into the community. It is to be hoped that the appointment of a co-ordinator of voluntary services (HMPS, 2000), which took effect from January 2001, will help to bridge the gap between prisons and the community. It should also help in reducing the number of prisoners held in isolation without damaging the high level of security that is in place at present (HMPS, 2000). This appointment is both an interesting and a brave initiative in prison service thinking: giving voluntary services a more formal and focused localised link with prisons is welcome for a number of reasons, not the least being the need for prisoners to mix with people outside the service as an essential part of their process of rehabilitation and resettlement. Healthcare could become an integrated continuum. Nurses may wish to consider a client whose release is imminent and think of the ways that they can exert leadership in this area.

When considering the culture of control, nurses could examine their own judgemental attitudes and the misuse of power. There are many insidious ways in which cruelty can be introduced into the relationship with inmates: for example, making a prisoner wait unnecessarily long for things, or making promises that are not kept. Having power and control is something that certain members of the prison staff enjoy – some actually come into the job for the satisfaction they get from controlling others, both prisoners and other members of staff. This is no different from the bullying found in other organisations. The services, teaching and hospitals are three examples of organisations where bullying goes on and has a devastating effect on people working in them (Norman *et al.*, 2001).

Some staff find the added power of being prominent members of a union a way in which they can stand out in the crowd, something they could never do if they were to be judged on the day-to-day quality of their work performance. Of course, there will always be a core of sensitive professionals whose talents and commitment can be built on to change the behaviour of the few who stand out.

Coon (1998) describes the importance of getting to know a little about other groups (no single culture has all the answers) as this can be personally rewarding and the insight gained can help to reduce friction and conflict. For managers, in particular, this is important. Organisations are managed through people, and it is essential that staff understand the long-term objectives of a service. In any organisation, people are the main asset and it is only sensible to make time for them. Inclusive leadership, allowing others to own and share vision and contribute their ideas to the running of a department will foster a sense of ownership and team spirit, as well as strong and healthy group dynamics.

It is also good management practice to deal with conflict both speedily and professionally. Conflict can be very positive if it is managed, but it can be devastating and destructive if it is left to fester; then it damages existing relationships and impedes progress. Often the best solution for conflict is compromise and this requires clear articulation and agreement. Once compromise is achieved goals can be attained. Most groups have a leader or spokesperson, and when problems arise, it is important to engage positively with the leader and other members of the group. In this way, it is hoped, conflicts can be resolved without alienating anyone.

Prior to the partnership arrangements, nurses working in a prison frequently worked in an isolated environment, where there was constant pressure to expand their scope of practice to meet new needs, demands and challenges. Their working environment can be both hostile and stressful. Areas of conflict can arise for a nurse working within the legal parameters of the nurse's Code of Professional Conduct (UKCC, 1992). For example, the strict handling of medicines and issues of confidentiality may not be fully understood or appreciated by non-colleagues. If nurses expect their colleagues to understand the role and function of nurses and their need to work within the Code of Professional Conduct, it is incumbent on them to spend some time explaining the concepts. Similarly, if nurses wish to know about the specialist skills and codes of practice of their colleagues they must learn to listen. Dialogue of this nature is important if conflicts are to be resolved and relationships built and maintained. It is professionally arrogant for people to join a service and expect others to understand, without explanation or discussion, their role, function and values. Nurses often forget that others do not understand their language and common assumptions.

Culture is a complex issue – it relates to membership of a family group, religious beliefs, social class, gender and ethnicity, as well as to work groups. It cannot be repeated enough that, in the work situation in particular, understanding of the culture is necessary if any success is to be achieved or any progress made.

Socialisation

Socialisation has been described as the process by which we learn how different groups work and individuals function within them (Malim & Birch, 1998). It is a lifelong process that helps us deal with new experiences. As a concept it is important to the nurse working within the prison culture because he or she is primarily working with prison officers, and may be socialised into their culture and possibly forget the values that underpin nursing. Equally, a prison officer working with a large group of nurses may be socialised into their type of behaviour without even being conscious of the process. Social behaviour is affected when people interact with each other (Coon, 1998). Each person in the interaction affects the behaviour of the other; the powers of conformity and compliance are strong in such dynamics.

Conformity and compliance

Conformity occurs when members of a group behave in a similar way to others in the group. Consider the enormous pressure on new members of staff to adapt. The power of the uniform and the prevailing attitudes of care in a clinical environment have significant impact upon how a new group member behaves. Once new entrants into a care setting have assessed the prevailing values, they are able to relax and join the group, developing a sense of belonging. When the dominant theme is difficult to pinpoint, they may be anxious until they can accurately identify the value system and the accepted way of behaving. The unconscious need to conform is so strong it can even affect how and what we eat (Norman *et al.*, 2001). The power of leadership is obvious here, and the message for prison healthcare is strong.

Compliance is a more complex concept. It occurs when members behave in the same way as the other members of the group, even when they may feel uncomfortable doing so. Consider the scapegoating of individuals that occurs. For instance, an influential leader is negative about the skills of a doctor and because of this the rest of the staff may respond in a negative manner and blame the doctor whenever anything goes wrong. Reverse the situation and consider how popularity is promoted and carries others along on a tide of contagious goodwill. The danger of compliance is that eventually a person may come to adopt the values that underpin the compliant behaviour. (Nurses might remember things that they felt resistant to when starting in prison hospital service that they now accept as part of the job.) Think how important this principle is: compliance, with peer pressure as a trigger, leads to conformity. These needs to conform and comply are powerful tools to utilise when trying to bring about change. Orientation programmes, briefings and debriefings, giving feedback on performance and offering alternative behaviours to undesirable conduct are all examples of the efforts made to bring about perceived desirable conformity and compliance. This emphasises the significance of mentoring and supervision. Also, encouraging new team members to keep reflective diaries and to give feedback to their groups highlights the issues and idiosyncrasies that stand out during a settling-in phase. These can then be discussed within the influences of group dynamics, which are subject to the members' needs to conform and comply.

Groups

Work groups are made up of individuals of all personality types, age ranges, gender, ethnic backgrounds, cultural diversity, skills, intelligence and values. Pennington (1986, p. 220) defines a group as 'involving at least three persons who communicate with one another to co-ordinate their activities in the pursuit of common goals'. He develops this definition by discussing groups under the headings of different roles, leadership, sets of norms and membership rules. Group members, then, can be said to:

- communicate and interact with each other
- come together to perform certain tasks or achieve goals.

Groups are structured so that individuals occupy roles, have status and power and conform, to some extent, to group norms. Members of a group have a sense of belonging to it and group members are independent, as they work towards shared goals. (Think about the different professional and social groups that you belong to and compare your motivation to be in each and the satisfaction that membership gives you. Note if you behave differently in each and consider the reason why, in terms of group influence. Then compare this with your working group.) Norms are the established behaviours of a group. There are uniformities in behaviour so that consistency between members occurs. Norms lead to group rules that are influenced by the group members who have status.

A great deal has been written about groups in social psychology and it is well worth reading one of the books from the reference section of this chapter and thinking through the issues.

Role

A role has been defined as 'a set of obligations and expectations' (Malim & Birch, 1998, p. 691). Pennington describes three assumptions about roles: expected role, perceived role and enacted role (Pennington, 1986, p. 226).

(1) Expected role is the behaviour others expect that the role holder should engage in.
(2) Perceived role is the way that the role holder thinks he or she should behave.
(3) Enacted role is the actual behaviour that the role holder engages in.

When these three are in harmony there are very few problems, but when there is disparity between the three role assumptions, members of a group will exert pressure to achieve conformity. Members of a healthcare group in a prison may play different roles. Compare the role of a prison officer with that of a nurse to find potential for conflict. Tremendous pressure may be put on a staff member to conform to an alien philosophy in the treatment of a prisoner; there can be differences in the behaviour of staff members, even in simple things like how an individual is addressed, or the type of response given to a simple and polite request from a prisoner. Thus, the role that we adopt in a group affects the way we communicate with others and the way in which others relate to us. However, the role of the leader is particularly important in a group, and can have a powerful social influence, which is a crucial theme in this chapter.

Attitudes

Attitudes are a strong component of social behaviour and have a huge influence upon the behaviour of social groups and individuals. One only has to think about the effect on group members of hearing that a new member soon to join the staff has a particular attitude with which they do not agree.

Attitudes have a strong emotional element. For instance, some of the offences that particular prisoners have committed can arouse very negative feelings. In the prison culture there may be certain offences that are viewed as trivial or even as having a certain heroism about them, while others, notably where offences against children are concerned, always trigger negative and often quite vengeful attitudes.

Attitudes are held by everybody about almost everything and they influence how we perceive others and the labels we put on them – whether we like, dislike or simply tolerate them. Significantly, they are often formed by cultural norms and are therefore an important consideration in the prison culture. Attitudes are also formed from direct experience. For instance, an attitude about a difficult or unpopular area of nursing may change significantly once someone has had a placement or the opportunity to work in that particular area of practice. (Good management is important in ensuring that correct messages about a clinical area are conveyed prior to placement.) Significantly for nurses, attitudes can be developed through role-modelling (Malim & Birch, 1998). Finally, understanding an issue can change perception and the formation of attitudes. For example, in a nursing conference the description of a client's childhood may provide an insight into the behaviour that led to conviction and explain some current behaviour, leading nurses to change their viewpoint from dislike and fear to empathy and understanding that enables them to deliver more appropriate care. As attitudes can be held unconsciously, the value of having a colleague observe you at work cannot be underestimated and it may be worthwhile visiting Chapter 5 'Enhancing Practice through Education', which addresses this issue.

Pennington (1986, p. 60) says that attitudes are relatively enduring but are also easy to change. Attitudes get us ready to respond in certain ways and help us to plan behaviour, for instance, coping with fear; this is often a real issue for nursing staff, either because of threats of aggression or because of violent incidents in their working environment. This is particularly so in accident and emergency departments, some areas of psychiatry, and regularly in prisons. Nurses become quite expert in facilitating the de-escalation of such incidents, and both authors have witnessed quite small and frail nurses resolving incidents in which the aggressors were enormous in comparison to them. This is a good example of an attitude being picked up by an aggressive person and interpreted as that of a professional at work, capable and competent, so that the nurse can produce positive outcomes from situations that, for whatever reason, are alive with anger, frustration and potential violence.

Attitudes are often described as having a three-part structure: *cognitive, affective* and *conative* (Pennington, 1986) – in other words thinking, feeling and acting. The thinking aspect of an attitude is supported by beliefs, such as believing that fat people are lazy, or that smokers are self-destructive. The feeling part of an attitude is the emotion or the evaluation that is provoked. Whether something is perceived as good or bad reflects a person's values. We may feel disgust that an overweight person is eating a cake, repulsed by the sight and smell of cigarette smoke. The acting or conative element is the behaviour that we engage in when confronted with the attitude; with the overweight people we might make a remark about calories or show intolerance to them at work. We may fan the air around people who are smoking or activate an aerosol spray in their vicinity, or even be verbally aggressive towards them. The three elements of an attitude are, on the whole, internally consistent and are learned aspects of our behaviour that make us behave in certain ways.

Pennington (1986) describes how people tend to develop the same attitudes to those people that they like and tend to seek out friends who share similar attitudes to their own. This is called the *adaptive* function. The *knowledge* function concerns the information we possess about the world, allowing us to feel safe and familiar with our surroundings and able to predict what might happen within the environment, both physical and social. These are important functions of orientation programmes. Pennington goes on to describe the *ego defence* function of attitudes, which is concerned with preserving our own self-esteem. Knowledge about the functions of attitudes can thus be seen to be important when working on changing attitudes. It is also useful to know that there is a consistency between the three elements that constitute an attitude.

Tackling this consistency by changing one element of a system of attitudes is an important way of systematically achieving attitude change. But achieving attitude change can be difficult. Given that attitudes have a three-part structure, cognitive, affective and conative, when more than one area is tackled the chances of achieving change are high. From this point of view, persuasion and reasoned argument are additional useful tools when trying to bring about changes.

Coon (1998) says that persuasion is more likely to be effective:

- when the persuader is likeable and trustworthy
- when the message appeals to emotions, especially fear and anxiety
- if personally desired results can be achieved, perhaps a reduction in anxiety
- if the message is backed by facts
- if the persuader has nothing to gain if the message is accepted
- when the message is repeated frequently.

Persuasion, then, is a powerful tool in altering attitudes (Coon, 1998, p. 681). Unless one changes a person's attitude, any change in behaviour is potentially isolated and not part of the larger learning process. A manager who instructs staff to make changes in behaviour may not change the underlying attitude. A manager who facilitates a change in attitude will see a range of changes taking place commensurate with the change in the value base. Persuasion rather than formal instruction is a much more effective agent for change. It is within the power of a manager with an appropriate leadership style to facilitate changes in attitudes. For example, exchanging views, modelling expert and correct behaviour and valuing caring may create cognitive dissonance within the team and provoke a need to conform in its members.

There is no doubt that expertise, trustworthiness and likeability influence the attitude formation of others (Coon, 1998). However, the characteristics of the recipient of persuasion are also significant, including intelligence, ability to understand the message, the damage to or strength of self-esteem, personality and flexibility. And it must be noted that the strength of using such techniques lies in planning them and thinking things through, rather than relying on luck.

The dynamics of change

It is impossible in such a chapter as this to consider the dynamics of a culture without paying due attention to the processes of change. Change theory is an important concept, and merits on its own a book devoted to nurses working in prisons; therefore, we would encourage reading around the subject as strategy is planned to develop a working culture. The following discussion is based on the authors' personal experiences of changes in organisations with which they have been involved during their careers.

First, it is essential that everyone in the team, as far as possible, can work out what changes need to be made and how it will be known that they have happened. Following this, reactions tend to occur in cycles. The first is a wave of enthusiasm during which everyone gets high on the agreed ideals being worked towards. A lot of energy goes into this phase, and it is important to maximise on this, to meet learning needs and to have a communications and feedback strategy.

Next comes a backlash wave of doubt: there are unexpected hitches and hiccups – perhaps the night staff have not been briefed; people start to feel tired and a bit beaten, or unsure that they have the skills needed to achieve an objective. (People may at this point think that it was better the way it was before.) To keep morale going, it is crucial during this stage to enable a leader to emerge, someone who has the confidence to deal with uncertainty, who predicts problems and caters for them with team meetings, reports, evaluations, encouragement. The significance of learning on the job cannot be over-emphasised, and clinical supervision is a crucial tool here too. Note that as there is both positive and negative learning it is important to have good role models to learn from. A nurse, of course, is required to maintain professional standards at all times and in all situations.

Then comes a period of maintenance. Here, it is necessary to keep the momentum going to manage the transition and to refine the process, gradually letting go of driving it once the changes have been internalised and accepted as the group norm. Within waves of change, there will always be significant personalities who emerge. For example, the enthusiasts, keen to start yesterday, may need help in slowing down and planning. They may drive some mad with their energy and have a degree of naivety about the resistance of others. At the other end of the continuum of commitment are the laggards who resist, get disgruntled and disaffected and need careful handling during a process they do not welcome. It is here that mixing personalities and maximising upon knowledge of attitudes, conformity and compliance can assist with skilful team-building. It is essential to respect all viewpoints and there is a lot that can be done to build on the energy generated by emotions. There is also the saboteur, the wolf in sheep's clothing who pretends to go along with new ideas but quietly raises doubts and undermines the confidence of others. Then there is the fence-sitter who cannot decide what to opt for. One way to deal with these various personalities is to discuss change at team meetings, but also to organise clinics away from the team where people can pop in and discuss their fears with the team leader in confidence and in private. It helps to retain a sense of humour, to have patience and, most important, to value and respect all viewpoints.

Conclusion

This chapter has addressed the power of the dynamics of working groups. Difficult dynamics, misunderstood compliance and poor socialisation have a direct impact upon the care that can be offered. They will also adversely affect team spirit (the corporate feel that is needed for a successful group to work) and the pleasure of being a team member. The essential basics of clinical supervision, mentorship and preceptorship – not only for the newly qualified but also for all staff new to an area – cannot be overvalued as powerful tools for achieving a strong and healthy culture. You may need to think about assertiveness and the behaviour that transmits this, the power of self-awareness, communication and relationship skills, and conflict management – it is hoped that this chapter will send you back to the library. Dealing with your personal development and seeing its impact upon your working culture is a dynamic and rewarding process.

References

Coon, D. (1998) *Introduction to Psychology: Exploration and Application*, 8th edn. Brooks/Cole, Pacific Grove, California, USA.

DOH (1992) *Report of the Committee of Inquiry into Complaints about Ashworth Hospital* (The Blom-Cooper Report). HMSO, London.

Hayes, N. & Orrell, S. (1993) *Psychology: An Introduction*, Ch. 20. Longman, London.

HMPS (2000) *Appointment of Voluntary Sector Co-Ordinator*. Press Release. HM Prison Service, Home Office, London.

Malim, T. & Birch, A. (1998) *Introductory Psychology*. Macmillan, London.

Norman, A., Parrish, A. & Birchenall, P. (2001) Not so happy at work. *Nurse Education Today*, **21**, 83–85.

Pennington, D.C. (1986) *Essential Social Psychology*. Edward Arnold, London.

UKCC (1992) *Code of Professional Conduct for the Nurse, Midwife and Health Visitor*, 3rd edn. United Kingdom Central Council for Nursing, Midwifery and Health Visiting, London.

Further reading

ANA (1995) *Scope and Standards of Nursing Practice in Correctional Facilities*. American Nurses Association, Washington, DC.

Ashworth Hospital Authority (1997) *The Written Submission of Ashworth Hospital Authority by the Committee of Inquiry into the Personality Disorder Unit*. Ashworth Hospital Authority, Ashworth.

Fallon, P., Bluglass, R., Edwards, B. & Daniels, G. (1999) *Report of the Committee of Inquiry into the Personality Disorder Unit, Ashworth Special Hospital*, Vol. 2, Expert evidence on personality disorder (The Fallon Report). The Stationery Office, London.

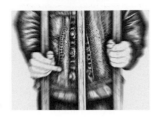

5 Enhancing Practice through Education

SALLY THOMSON

It is often said that there are three important factors to consider when developing a workforce – education, education, education. The need for education of prisoners has been emphasised by politicians, governors and prisoner support groups, but it is also true for prison staff and not least prison nurses. This chapter describes the essential need for nurses to update their professional skills, and provides some useful and practical ways of doing this.

Introduction

Regardless of the roles nurses carry out in prison nursing, whether as specialists in preventive health, carers of patients with thought disorders and mood changes or carers of adults in ill health, they are, in common with all registered nurses, midwives and health visitors, responsible for their own learning and professional development and the learning and professional development of others.

The mandatory requirements for post-registration education and practice (PREP) place nurses firmly in the arena of lifelong learning. Lifelong learning will ensure that a nurse's practice is contemporary and the best it can be. When a prison health service is geared towards providing a learning environment within its organisation, professional education can take place in individual clinical areas.

The reader, whether learning simply for pleasure or working towards an academic award, will find that this chapter will:

- describe the features of lifelong learning
- discuss the principles of a learning culture
- outline the educational requirements of PREP
- detail the differing ways that learning needs can be met
- briefly discuss the significance of learning styles
- consider factors that affect learning.

The chapter is designed to be an enjoyable and tailor-made way of learning and to assist the transference of new learning into practice.

Lifelong learning

The term 'lifelong learning' has come into popularity since the Dearing Report on higher education (National Committee of Inquiry into Higher Education, 1997). The principle behind the notion is that if all individuals take responsibility for their own development it will create a 'learning society'. The report hopes that people from all walks of life will continue with training and education in order to keep abreast of rapid change in the world, at work and in their lives. The report is focused upon higher education but the concept of lifelong learning is envisaged in its expectations that universities will:

- enable economic competitiveness
- support the richness of our culture
- foster the values of a cohesive, democratic and pluralistic society.

The overt message in the report is that we all need to learn all our lives (nurses may have thoughts about the constant development and updating needed to maintain their knowledge and nursing expertise, while the rate of change and development in health is so rapid). In the context of prison healthcare, the values and skills that underpin nursing care may already have been seriously challenged by the culture within which nurses are working (Norman & Parrish, 1999).

Learning can present itself in many guises, from lengthy formal courses with an academic credit rating to a single day spent with an expert practitioner. Merely solving problems at work can be a learning experience. Regardless of the means that are adopted, learning may increase confidence and self-esteem and at times of stress it may maintain personal morale. Learning is an active process. It works best when it is planned and requires the learner to categorise and order thoughts.

The ability to initiate and keep abreast of change also depends upon learning, which ensures that an individual remains flexible, open, questioning and able to evaluate a challenge. Edwards (1997), in a challenging chapter on lifelong learning, discusses the power that this activity can bring. He quotes Foucault:

> Knowing if one can think differently than one thinks and perceive differently than one sees is absolutely necessary if one is to go on looking and reflecting at all ...
>
> (Foucault, 1987, p. 8, cited in Edwards, 1997)

Lifelong learning provides the philosophy that underpins the re-registration requirements. One thing is certain, it is not too soon for any nurse to be working towards those requirements now!

Creating a learning culture

While it is important that PREP meets personal needs, nurses may find that as a team they have a shared wish to learn and develop. By pooling their learning they may be able to develop a common framework to enhance the care that they give. A group approach to PREP will allow sharing of resources and talents, pooling of ideas and the development of a strong nursing and group identity within the prison culture. If a team identifies learning needs according to shared criteria, for example, a role description, or shared values about nursing, a strong sense of purpose may develop linked to future action. The team may increase its understanding, reduce the workload associated with learning, and effectively solve challenging nursing problems. In time, as confidence grows within the group it may feel able to make the learning culture multi-disciplinary. Certainly it can create an efficient way of learning directly applicable to current care. Learning as a group may increase the effectiveness and economy of the activity, and it will allow for social support and feed into purposeful change.

A few words of caution though. A team approach is a positive way forward, but, in the beginning, do not try to do too much (the section on ways of learning and learning styles later in the chapter has some obvious messages). It is important to consider the dynamics of the working group, taking in members' responses to this team approach idea. Communication, tolerance, dominance and deviance all need to be catered for within the group. Ground rules may help the group achieve its task and cope with problems. Rotating the chair is also useful and can be a learning experience in its own right. Consideration should be given to confidentiality and psychological safety within the group. And one final point in this note of caution – it is important to retain the spirit of PREP, which is about individuals and their learning, not about assessment of one individual against the perceived performance of others.

But now a note of encouragement – a group model of learning can be a powerful and enjoyable way of updating; it can take the stress out of PREP, and it can contribute towards a learning culture.

Educational requirements to maintain registration

The post-registration education and practice requirements (PREP) affect every nurse, midwife and health visitor who wishes to stay on the NMC (Nursing and Midwifery Council) register. When practitioners register with the NMC they are confirming that they have maintained the requirements for PREP, yet many practitioners at all levels and in all families of nursing feel anxious and worried about the process (see below). PREP is about developing individual nurses, midwives and health visitors in order to improve standards of patient and client care (UKCC, 1997). It is about developing standards through deeper insight and understanding and is achieved through planned professional development. PREP requires practitioners to do four things to maintain registration:

(1) every three years, re-register by completing a notification to practice form (changes in practice, for instance, dual registration, require notification)
(2) undertake a minimum of five study days, or equal activity, every three years
(3) maintain a personal professional profile containing details of professional development
(4) undertake a return to practice programme that is approved by the statutory body if practice time falls below 750 hours or 100 working days in five years.

Study days and the maintenance of the professional profile concern the majority of nurses. These aspects will be developed in the next sections. The UKCC document *PREP and You* (1997), sent to all registered nurses, is a useful and easy read (this can be found in all nursing libraries and probably in most clinical areas).

Five study days

PREP requires that five study days, or their equivalent, be undertaken every three years. This can be interpreted broadly and creatively and dovetailed to learning needs. PREP is not designed to push nurses towards formal courses of study, but for some it will be the final encouragement to do so. The requirement is designed to help develop practice and skills at a level and pace that suits practitioners' current needs. Five days equates to approximately 35 hours of study. This 'study' is open to broad interpretation and thus can be readily manipulated to meet needs. For instance, a conference on suicide may be just the thing needed to update the skills required to deal with depressed, suicidal people. This acquisition of a new and deepened knowledge base may inspire practitioners (such as prison nurses) to learn how to apply this insight to their roles within the cultures in which they operate. A conference then, or a traditional study day, may be a wise investment in practitioners' development, and may inspire follow-up trips to the library at a university or medical school to conduct focused literature searches on aspects of care. Active reading and note-taking is a valid updating activity that can be applied to practice. For prison nurses, a literature search may provoke questions and raise issues that may be resolved by spending a day with a clinical nurse specialist in this field, in either a prison or a secure environment, or ways may be found to turn theory into practice with the benefit of other nurses' experiences.

When interests have thus been aroused, nurses may wish to explore issues with other health workers: reading may highlight ethical aspects and inspire nurses to seek the advice of an ethicist; exploring the use of complementary therapies may lead to contacts with nurses who use complementary techniques in their practice. By the time the issues have been reflected upon, and different practical learning opportunities have been undertaken, 35 hours of learning will be in the bank. All that needs to be done is to make a documentary record, including objectives achieved/intended with this learning. This documentation will now be available should the NMC wish to audit a practitioner, but it should also prove useful in improving practice.

To summarise, then, study can be interpreted as:

- a workshop or study day
- a literature search usefully applied to practice
- a focused visit to another area
- time spent with another practitioner with different skills and expertise
- the use of distance learning material
- a taught course
- a professional debate (for example the Royal College of Nursing Congress and its fringe events).

The formula for updating is first that it has significance to practitioners and their practice. But a word of caution: many people have jumped on the PREP bandwagon as a means of generating income – most study activities offer a quality learning experience but some do not. Examine carefully any marketing material that is trying to entice you to pay for something – points, certificates or study days are not compulsory as a means or proof of learning. PREP is about self-verification – demonstrating that what practitioners have done meets their own needs. Finally, in this note of caution, there are times in everyone's life when learning is both exciting and rewarding. PREP maximises on this principle of intrinsic motivation; however, there are also times when the need to achieve updating is the final straw in a pile of stresses. PREP allows practitioners to do the best that they can in their own areas; it relies on them being honest with themselves about whether they are just scoring up the hours or whether they are developing themselves and their practice. Beware of comparisons with others that leave feelings of vulnerability; it is the quality of practitioners' own practice that they are accountable for – that is the key to learning.

The professional profile

The UKCC (1997, p. 11) suggested that there are six stages to professional development that are logical and easy to follow, although they have been modified for use here.

(1) Review of competence
     — identify strengths
     — identify weaknesses
     — designate areas of weakness to be worked on for a period of, say, two to five years.
(2) Set learning objectives
     — note what is to be achieved
     — state how achievement will be recognised
     — set a time limit (useful to prevent taking on too much).
(3) Develop an action plan
     — decide on strategies to meet objectives
     — determine if a facilitator is available if required
     — seek any necessary funding
     — ensure feedback on progress.
(4) Implement the plan
     — it may be necessary at this stage to seek support from management regarding off duty, study time, funding, etc.
(5) Evaluate learning
     — have objectives been achieved?
     — were there benefits for the client group?

—   how will the new learning be disseminated to peer groups?
(6)   Record study time and learning outcomes in the profile.

When registering with the NMC a practitioner will be asked to confirm that a professional profile has been maintained. The practitioner may be requested to produce this, as part of the mechanism to ensure the quality of PREP. Before moving on to discuss the development of profiles it may be helpful to distinguish between portfolios and professional profiles.

Portfolios are collections of evidence that are unique to given individuals. They can be multifarious collections containing almost anything (such as statements on why nursing was chosen as a career, held values or personal relationships). This 'hard evidence' is often kept in a box or old suitcase in the loft, possibly of parents' houses – contracts, photos, career memorabilia, some certificates, badges, old essays, leaving cards, diaries, journals, a curriculum vitae (CV) – the list can be extensive. Going through these may trigger memories (for instance, what influenced the direction that a career took). Of course, not all personal information is stored in portfolios, some is contained only in the head, while more may be stored in employees' personnel files – significant feedback in appraisals, life events, clinical incidents – all or some of which may have triggered a change in thinking about the delivery of care or possibly changed or developed a career. A portfolio, then, is a 'collection of evidence that demonstrates learning' (Hinchliff, 1999, p. 105) and in its broadest sense it is a collection that reflects professional life, although aspects of it may be private and personal. As mentioned in Chapter 3, in 2000 the Prison Health Task Force introduced a nursing portfolio for all nursing team members including non-registered professionals. There is now a clear expectation that all members of the healthcare team provide evidence of professional updating.

A profile is a more focused document. It may well be that a portfolio will provide five or six themes that dominate professional and career development to date and for which a set of objectives and a strategy for PREP study time could be extracted. These themes may provide the backbone of a profile. A profile, then, is 'a collection of information that gives details for the individual concerned for a particular purpose' (Hinchliff, 1999, p. 105) and it is the professional aspects of an individual that have been chosen to be made public. As such, it is the representation of the individual that exists in written form. Profiles can be used in ways other than for NMC requirements. They provide a tailor-made source of information for job applications, and can alert new colleagues and others to an individual's passions and interests in care. However, a profile is flexible and can be tailored to suit different audiences and for PREP requirements it provides the reflective framework of an individual. It is something that will need regular updating and development as experience and insight change the individual practitioner.

Profiles then are meant to enhance professional development, with the onus placed firmly on practitioners to portray themselves honestly – only they will know if they have done this. Constantly working on a profile can help practitioners to evaluate the significance of experience and may propel them into taking academic credits that help with the attainment of further academic qualifications.

Some practitioners might not know how to start a profile. They could begin by looking at their current role description. However, many of these are 'mature' descriptions that may need refining to reflect accurately the actual work done; some things may be out of date or have changed and developed since the post was first taken up.

From the role description, it is advisable for practitioners to focus on specific areas that they may realistically develop in the foreseeable future (for example, communicating with clients, giving expert care in a specific area, teaching others or maintaining safety). These should be noted as learning objectives for intended formal or informal study. Then a list of learning experiences for the past three to four years can be drawn up. These could be recorded under separate headings: for instance:

- courses that are given an academic rating (CATS – credit accumulation and transfer points), these include pre-registration programmes, modules, certificates, diplomas, or degrees, short courses and workshops
- learning undertaken to meet the requirements of PREP, that is, the learning that has affected practice and that has been reflected upon and developed as it has been tied into experience
- learning for learning's sake: the self-generated learning that we all do.

The UKCC determined five broad categories to demonstrate the range of learning that can be explored and used to plan development:

(1)   patient/client and colleague support (from mentorship to supervision of colleagues and support of clients)
(2)   care enhancement (new approaches to care, implications of standards)
(3)   practice development (research or visits)
(4)   reducing risk (health promotion and health and safety issues)
(5)   educational development.

They stressed that these provide a loose framework only, and are flexible in their interpretation by practitioners (UKCC, 1997). To complete this part of the profile, practitioners may log against each piece of learning (not that there will be reams of it) the aspects related to their role descriptions and mark areas where they have future enhancement plans, for example, complex skills, greater confidence or changed awareness. Some of this information may not be written down or may be in store somewhere not easily accessible, and it may only be identified as relevant to practitioners in bits and pieces over time. Writing and recording in profiles must be done in the practitioners' own style. Although the steps mentioned above may help, this activity may initially feel clumsy and false; perseverance, however, will bring about the development of style, and the profile should become a tool that will help practitioners to focus.

Profiles are also useful for professional appraisal sessions, helping in the identification/agreement of learning needs. In group meetings they can facilitate the sharing of reflections, help diagnose learning needs for units or teams and assist in the identification and promotion of individual skills.

The activity of developing a profile should not take too long, but may involve practitioners coming and going from it as ideas occur. But as they develop their profiles they will be taking part in lifelong learning, the theme of this chapter. (It may be worth carrying a small notebook around, as ideas tend to pop up at the strangest times and in the unlikeliest places.)

The format of profiles is something that should be given some thought. Some are on discs and easily adaptable; others can be bought as pre-designed documents. But make sure they will serve the purpose. Many pre-formatted documents start with the details that form a CV. Practitioners must evaluate whether they want this style imposed upon them. Some use a notebook or loose sheets in an A4 file. It may be a good idea to experiment with a couple of approaches before investing in a glossy profile that gathers dust on a shelf. The joy of a profile is that it is a self-painted snapshot, but it is a live snapshot that must reflect the present, being continuously brought up to date.

A shelf is not a good storage place. As a profile is a personal tool, a manager has no right to see it and comment, especially if this document is used to keep reflective accounts that if read by somebody else would breach confidentiality. Therefore the safe-keeping of profiles is essential. If profiles are called for audit by the NMC then reflective accounts must be edited to prevent confidentiality breaches.

Using reflection to meet the requirements of PREP

The processes suggested to put a profile together are reflective in nature and they are designed to help practitioners maximise on experience as part of ongoing professional development. Using a framework may help practitioners to get into the habit of using this reflective technique. Its use can be particularly help-ful when nurses begin to write or discuss accounts of significant experiences in order to learn from them, or to de-brief individuals after an outburst or some critical event that has happened in a care situation. Developing the technique can make its use automatic, assisting an individual not only to use it to make more sense out of life but to become, with little effort, a reflective practitioner. Additionally, it may be a successful way of facilitating professional develop-ment in peer groups. Incidentally, written accounts are more valid as they can be re-visited to see how it was, rather than how it was remembered!

Boud *et al.* (1985) have devised a model that is helpful for reflection. It is divided into three stages: the experience, the reflective process and outcomes. Let us explore a situation in which a nurse has been manipulated by a patient and feelings of anger follow. To begin, reflect on the incident, recording the key points exactly as they happened from the nurse's point of view. Next, it is important to identify the feelings that went with the event – manipulative clients often use flattery: for example, the client may have disclosed some details or feelings that made the nurse feel both helpful and supportive. (When manipula-tion is happening successfully we are rarely aware that it is going on – otherwise we would put a stop to it.) To start off, the nurse has a lack of awareness and insight, but when on reflection it is realised that the nurse has been manipulated, frustration and anger follow.

Reflection is an important stage in the learning process. Schönn (1987) describes how reflection helps others to make decisions in conditions of uncer-tainty. He describes two ways of undertaking this: first, by thinking back on an action and, second, by stopping before an action or in mid-action to take stock and devise an alternative outcome. (Stopping mid-action may be useful for the nurse when self-monitoring but it has implications when a nurse stops a col-league. If it is found necessary to stop the ongoing practice of a colleague then a nurse must preserve the dignity and feelings of credibility of the practitioner and offer feedback and a way forward out of earshot.)

Changing course mid-action in a nursing situation can become as normal as changing direction in a car; once the principles of driving are understood and practised, driving becomes an automatic skill. Ability to change mid-action is a necessary skill in improving the quality of nursing care.

To return to the client situation, the nurse reflecting on the situation may feel embarrassed about the fact that colleagues are aware of the mistake made, or may feel justified in taking negative action against the client or just remain cross with the whole situation.

To prevent these negative outcomes it is important for the nurse to look for positive emotions. The fact can be emphasised that the nurse did realise at some stage that manipulation had taken place. The nurse can have the satisfaction of knowing that he or she has developed insight and has learned something.

At this third phase of the model, the nurse can write down the new understanding about the behaviour that this patient uses when being manipulative. Being able to recognise the signs is a result of reflecting mid-action. Further, the nurse may rehearse strategies for assertive responses to stop the unwanted behaviour and, realising how difficult this person must be for more junior colleagues to cope with, may consider how best to arrange for care to be delivered so that no single nurse becomes overwhelmed with stress and emotion. In retrospect, manipulative behaviour has become a rich resource for learning, considering support for colleagues and the delivery of care.

Such reflection on nursing care may take place during study time for PREP when the nurse is evaluating experiences and the relevance of them for practice. It becomes a useful tool for making sense of all sorts of issues and is excellent as a technique for supporting others. The process quickly becomes internalised and automatic in its use, but until then it is a good idea to practise going through each stage of the process. (If such cases are to be cited in a profile then anonymity of clients and colleagues must be ensured.)

Using the right type of learning to meet objectives

Learning theories can be simplistically divided into four main theories:

(1) cognitive, where new material has to be mentally processed to develop understanding – significant for health workers to enable them to see the place of learning in the delivery of care
(2) behavioural, where training, feedback and practice can develop a skill
(3) social, where we learn from the behaviour and learning of others
(4) experiential, which links loosely with the reflective issues already discussed above.

It is naive to think that each school of learning stands alone in professional development. We know from learning to drive that instructors are highly proficient in developing skills in others, but how much easier clutch control seems once you understand what is happening to the engine. Similarly, we may admire a person's leadership style but be unable to adopt such a style for ourselves until we understand the principles lying behind that style and are able to see how we can adopt them for our own use. But Biggs and Moore point out that learning is also affected by our personality, as well as by personal preferences and dislikes (Biggs & Moore, 1993).

Cognitive learning

Cognitive psychologists believe that the mental processing of thoughts helps us to learn: that learning requires accurate perception of information and the ability to store it and retrieve it from memory. Past experience and memory will interact with new learning to help make sense of it and to store it accurately in the memory bank. As cognitive processes mature over the years, it is worth remembering that clients with a learning disability may need teaching that is appropriate to the stage to which their learning ability has developed.

Biggs and Moore (1993, p. 102) describe *deep* and *surface* learning. An example of surface learning is the rote learning of a passage: this can be easily done without understanding and many of us can still quote text learned many years ago at school. Deep learning, in comparison, is 'plugged in' (Biggs & Moore, 1993, p. 312): on completion of a learning task, students will possess a great deal of knowledge about the content of the subject, they will be able to use the information in different situations, enjoy the process of learning and be prepared to invest time and effort in learning.

Principles can be extracted from Biggs and Moore's concept of deep learning and utilised when planning our own or others' learning situations. For example, we might use past experience and learning as pegs on which to hang new information, or move from known and familiar ideas to new and challenging ones. A study day designed without a theme, and with sessions placed randomly together, does not maximise on this principle. Then again, if students see the relevance of the knowledge that is being imparted, the need to learn may be appreciated. For example, a session on post-operative care for the prison nurse may not be as relevant as managing challenging and unsocial behaviour. Cognitive learning works well when there is interaction with others as part of the process of learning. Finally, learning is an active process: sitting and listening is only effective for short periods of time.

Behavioural learning

This type of learning consists of the shaping of behaviour towards a desired goal (Hinchliff, 1999). Connections made between stimulus and response are reinforced. Think of the patterns of behaviour evoked on hearing a 'violent incident' alarm. Many practitioners working with clients who require a high degree of skilled teaching will be familiar with behavioural theories,

and nurses who have undergone training will have been taught using rein-
forcement techniques – succeeding at a task becomes rewarding and the
lesson is thus reinforced. If a task, such as injection technique, is broken
down into small steps, the student's success is guaranteed and the technique
itself becomes rewarding as an acquired skill.

Some principles emerge from behavioural theories that are important for
structuring learning (Hinchliff, 1999):

- each step in the learning process should be short and emerge from previously learned behaviours
- learning should be regularly rewarded and the reward should occur immediately after the desired behaviour has occurred.

Rewards can range from affirmations, nods and smiles to outright praise. However, even when learning alone, the intrinsic feedback of success will reinforce
new skills, for instance, mastering the skills of information technology.

Within behavioural learning strategies there are all sorts of learning and development opportunities, ranging from people skills, such as practising confronta-
tions, to technical skills, such as assisting with lumbar punctures.

Social learning

Social learning theories overlap, to a large extent, with behavioural and cognitive theories, but the power of this approach is obvious when unconscious or
vigorous learning is demonstrated, for example, when a practitioner is confronted with a situation and uses skills that have unconsciously been picked up
from another. It is learning by watching the behaviour of others and observing
the consequences it produces for them (Atkinson *et al.*, 1996). However, learning by deliberately modelling behaviour on that of others is planned and conscious; complex patterns of behaviour can be developed in this way (Quinn,
1995). Myles (1993) holds that emotional responses can be learned in this way.
(It may be useful for you to stop and think of a role model who has significantly
influenced you. That person is likely to be responsible for an enormous amount
of vigorous learning on your part. Even more daunting to consider is the influence that you may have had on the behaviour of others!)

This model is interesting when deviance is explored. Research indicates that
most influential role models are seen by others as having status (Melia, 1983;
Fretwell, 1985). Bandura (1977) identifies four features of social learning
theory that may be utilised in learning plans.

(1)   Attentional processes, or the degree of liking between the role model and the observer and how distinctive and useful the observed behaviour is. The observer has to come into frequent contact with the model to increase the chances of learning. Also, the observer has to be aroused and able to make sense of what is happening. It is obvious that the accuracy of perception is important, and this can be supported with explanations by, questioning of and discussions with the role model. The role model may enhance learning by alerting the observer to specific strategies or behaviours.

(2)   Retention processes, or remembering. This is crucial and is helped by rehearsal and repetition.

(3)   Motor reproduction, or the enactment of the observed behaviour. This needs to be evaluated in terms of accuracy.

(4)   Motivation, or the meaning of the behaviour for the learner. If the behaviour is valued it is more likely to be learned.

Much social learning is unconscious. However, there are things that can be done to maximise upon the principles – shadowing someone, choosing a suitable role model, raising awareness of the behaviour observed, discussing strategies with the role model, etc. – and the learning that is on offer will then be overt. Importantly, writing down observations quickly will enhance memory. If motivation is zero the observer is unlikely to benefit from such opportunities.

Experiential learning

The distinction between personal learning, reflection and social learning is blurred, but there are ways to develop and meet the requirements for PREP by using an experiential cycle to process thoughts. This tool may be helpful when learning in peer groups that are trying to find shared meaning, perhaps when they are reorganising or delivering care in a different way. For practitioners working on their own it may be that the reflective model offers a framework that can be used independently. However, the distinguishing feature of the experiential cycle is that in each of the stages there is sharing of thoughts and perceptions.

These four ways of approaching learning (cognitive, behavioural, social and experiential) are not independent of each other, but practitioners may wish to reflect on the principles of each and consider which one will best meet their needs as they pursue their objectives for PREP and seek opportunities to do this. However, this also needs to be complemented by a consideration of preferred learning styles.

Maximising upon learning styles

How we learn depends upon how we learned to learn and we all do that in different ways. Honey and Mumford (Stengelhofen, 1996) describe four types of learning style: the activist, the reflector, the pragmatist and the theorist.

The *activist* enjoys new experiences, challenges and change, learns by processing thoughts and ideas with others and enjoys being centre stage. The *reflector* in contrast learns by reflecting before making choices, tends to learn from listening to the debate held by others and enjoys working alone. The *pragmatist* links theory with practice, uses problem-solving methods and is concerned to develop practical skills. The *theorist* thrives on theory and concepts, uses problem-solving to make sense of complex issues and benefits from learning in a structured way and linking in to theories.

It can be seen from the four styles that individuals will benefit from different learning opportunities and will even read and use this book in different ways. Maslin-Prothero (1997) describes ways in which different learning styles can be adopted, but at this stage in their careers learners may be advised to seek opportunities that make the most of their particular learning style. Practitioners may wish to log in their profiles the learning styles that best suit them.

Factors affecting learning

Embarrassment, discomfort, tiredness, pain and hunger all affect our ability to learn. Additionally, motivation influences learning, and interest is a key factor. It is therefore important when learning independently to recognise achievement and to keep a balance with any other commitments and interests. Anxiety affects learning – for example, trying to master a technical skill in front of colleagues who are viewed as powerful. Being worried or insecure in a learning situation may affect the ability to absorb or make sense of new material. Personality affects the process of learning (Honey & Marson, 1982). An extrovert may enjoy learning in a situation with frequent breaks and distractions, whereas such interruptions would put off a more introverted person.

From the above discussion, we can gather that learners should be sensible about the commitments that are made to learning, be in the right mood and have realistic expectations.

Evidence-based practice

The nature of this chapter does not allow for a significant input on evidence-based practice; however, the philosophy of learning supported by reflection underpins and forms the foundations of this crucial approach to care. A journal editorial (Editorial, 1998) describes evidence-based nursing as giving quantitative or qualitative meaning to the cause, course, diagnosis, treatment and economics of healthcare problems. Evidence-based nursing also allows quality assurance and continuing professional development.

Hinchliff (1999) describes how practising nursing using evidence requires skills in assessing, analysis, decision-making and reflection. She states that evidence-based practice can bridge the gap between theory and practice. Collecting nursing evidence to support care is a relatively new activity in the context of prison nursing. The service needs to rely and adapt evidence from other disciplines and families of nursing until its research body is developed. However, the principles of practising from an evidence base can do much to support a learning culture.

Conclusion

This chapter has discussed the concept of lifelong learning and placed it within the requirements that have to be fulfilled to remain on the professional register. Consideration has been given to the fostering of a learning organisation and the different approaches to learning that can be adopted. Learning styles and reflective processes have been considered as a way of tailoring learning activity to individual needs, and a strategy offered for the development of a professional profile.

Now it is time for you to consider all the different dimensions and have a go. Enjoy!

References

Atkinson, R.L., Atkinson, R.C., Smith, E., Ben, D. & Noten-Hokeksena, P. (1996) *Introduction to Psychology*, 12th edn. Harcourt Brace Jovanovich, New York.

Bandura, A. (1977) *Social Learning Theory*. Hall, New Jersey.

Biggs, J. & Moore, P. (1993) *The Process of Learning*, 3rd edn. Prentice Hall, London.

Boud, D., Keogh, R. & Walker, D. (1985) *Reflection: Turning Experience into Learning*. Kogan Page, London.

Editorial (1998) Evidence-based practice. *Evidence-Based Practice*, 1(1), 7–8.

Edwards, R. (1997) *Changing Places? Flexibility, Lifelong Learning and a Learning Society*. Routledge, London.

Fox, D.J. (1979) *Fundamentals of Research in Nursing*, 4th edn. Appleton Century Crofts, New York.

Fretwell, J. (1985) *Freedom to Change – the Creation of the Ward Learning Environment*. Royal College of Nursing, London.

Hinchliff, S. (ed.) (1999) *The Practitioner as Teacher*, 2nd edn. Bailliere Tindall, London.

Honey, P. & Marson, S.N. (1982) Ward sister – teacher or facilitator? An investigation into the behavioural characteristics of effective ward teachers. *Journal of Advanced Nursing*, 7, 347–57.

Maslin-Prothero, S. (1997) *Bailliere's Study Skills for Nurses*. Bailliere Tindall, London.

Melia, K. (1983) Students' views of nursing and being professional. *Nursing Times*, **79**(22), 28–30.

Myles, A. (1993) Psychology and healthcare. In *Nursing Practice and Healthcare*, (eds S.M. Hinchliff, S. Norman, & J. Schober). 2nd edn. Edward Arnold, London.

National Committee of Inquiry into Higher Education (1997) *Higher Education in the Learning Society* (The Dearing Report). HMSO, London.

Norman, A. & Parrish, A. (1999) Behind closed doors. *Nursing Standard*, **13**(45), 61.

Quinn, F.M. (1995) *The Principle and Practice of Nurse Education*, 3rd edn. Croom Helm, London.

Schönn, D.A. (1987) *Educating the Reflective Practitioner*. Jossey Bass, San Francisco.

Stengelhofen, J. (1996) *Teaching Students in Clinical Settings*. Chapman Hall, London.

UKCC (1997) *PREP and You*. United Kingdom Central Council for Nursing, Midwifery and Health Visiting, London.

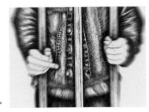

6 Educational Developments of the Nursing Team

LES STOREY

This chapter provides a description of the competence framework in the prison service, underpinned by the government's modernising health agenda. The author discusses the work of *Nursing in Secure Environments* (UKCC & University of Central Lancashire, 1999), and its impact upon training for prison nursing. He sets out a plan for the future training of the nursing workforce, and the associated benefits for the workforce and for patient care.

Introduction

The competence of the workforce is at the heart of a number of policy statements that will have an impact on prison healthcare over the next few years. *Nursing in Prisons* (DOH, 2000a) supports the development and implementation of competence-based models of education and development as identified in *Making a Difference* (DOH, 1999a) and *Fitness for Practice* (UKCC, 1999a) for the development of healthcare staff within the England and Wales prison service. The competence-based approach relies on a framework of competences that can be used to develop job descriptions and training programmes.

'Competences' are the knowledge, skills, abilities and behaviours that employees need to perform their work and that are the key levers for achieving results that will enable the organisation to achieve its healthcare objectives.

A 'competence framework' is a set of competences and includes associated behaviours that link directly to overall strategic priorities and the work that needs to be done to achieve them, as well as to levels of proficiency for each behaviour. The framework provides the proficiency levels and behaviours required for a specific job or class of job. A competence framework applies to a specific employee or population of employees. It can cover employees in a group of positions/jobs within a department, or employees belonging to a functional community. Frameworks can be applied in order to:

- recruit and select new staff
- develop appropriate induction programmes
- monitor and evaluate individual and team performance
- identify specific training and development needs
- develop training programmes to meet organisational, individual and team needs.

All of these are precursors to enabling practitioners to embrace lifelong learning as a concept for continuing professional development. The new emphasis on clinical governance, and the basis of *The Mental Health National Service Framework* (DOH, 2000b), strongly reinforces the principle that lifelong learning should be designed to meet organisational needs, as well as the individual expectations and aspirations of contributing professionals. This principle also applies within the prison service as healthcare provision partnerships develop with NHS providers.

The National Health Service Executive, in its health service circular *A First Class Service* (DOH, 1998), identified a number of proposals that were intended to support the delivery of a consistent and better quality service to patients. These were classified in the following way:

- the setting of clear national quality standards through the national service frameworks and the National Institute for Clinical Excellence (NICE)
- effective local delivery of quality clinical services: to be channelled through the concept of clinical governance, reinforced by a new statutory duty, and supported by programmes of lifelong learning and local delivery of professional self-regulation
- accurate and effective monitoring of the delivery of standards: to take place in the form of a new statutory commission for health improvement superimposed on an NHS performance assessment framework.

Organisations need competent staff, and competence frameworks go a long way to providing an empirical framework for embracing many of the concepts listed previously. Innovations and novel ideas in continuing professional development are being seen in a number of areas within forensic mental health and prison services. Professional development and clinical governance are tending to focus on certain criteria. Development should:

- be participative, with the focus on involving the practitioner
- be targeted towards direct patient care
- be aimed at meeting an identified educational need
- be based on accurate evidence that is educationally effective
- be lodged within the wider organisational strategic and development plans
- transfer across professional and service delivery boundaries
- reflect previous knowledge and experience of practice.

The fundamental aspects of programmes of continuing professional development revolve around the requirement that they should meet the professional needs of people together with their individual aspirations, but these have to be integrated with the needs of the services and their clients.

The implications of the above initiatives for the prison service and the pressure in the forthcoming years will be to ensure that the practical aspects of introducing these changes are in place. These will include:

- an adequate capacity of new technology and distance learning material that will maximise the way in which professional development is integrated with clinical governance
- identified expertise within professional and statutory bodies that will best support local professional development within the context of clinical governance
- an identified role for monitoring, peer review and appraisal in determining the structure of continuing professional development programmes
- an educational infrastructure within every health organisation that is designed to identify, analyse and meet the needs of its professional staff.

Education providers, at both pre- and post-registration, need to work more closely with service providers to ensure that programmes evolve that meet the needs of the nursing staff to work in these challenging and complex services. A competence-based approach offers some hope of a flexible and adaptable framework that can encompass many of the aspects under consideration. Full use should be made of existing programmes in the health, social and criminal justice sectors, and in addition energies should be directed at formulating more focused programmes.

Meeting patients' needs

The provision of more effective services that respond to the health needs of the prison population was at the heart of the report *The Future Organisation of Prison Health Care* (DOH, 1999b), which recommended the redesign and reshaping of healthcare in prisons and the inclusion of the health needs of the local prison population in local health authorities' planning and resource allocation. The report also identified the need to undertake health needs assessments of prisoners and to use the outcomes for developing the skills and competences of healthcare staff.

The report *Nursing in Secure Environments* (UKCC and University of Central Lancashire, 1999), which was the first major review of nursing undertaken in this sector, identified that the competences required for nurses working in secure environments are not clearly articulated by their employers. In a significant majority of cases, the job descriptions for nursing posts described the main components of the job, including lines of responsibility, but did not identify specific competences; this, however, is a failure identified across most of nursing, not just prison healthcare. Generic job descriptions do not help in defining and developing specific roles to meet particular health needs. As the prison services undertake health needs assessments, competence-based approaches would make it possible to match particular healthcare needs of prisoners with the skills of the healthcare team.

The job descriptions viewed as part of the UKCC secure environments project (UKCC & University of Central Lancashire, 1999) may be described as generic: they could apply to a wide range of posts in acute settings or in secure settings. Generic job descriptions do not provide the postholder with a framework for her/his continuing development or evaluate the effectiveness of an individual's practice. A small number of organisations are developing competence-based job descriptions using competence frameworks from a number of sources.

The general development of competences in the UK

Much work has been undertaken in the last few years to develop competences or national occupational standards for professionals. Competences can now be found in accountancy, engineering, psychology, social work, probation, health promotion and professions allied to medicine.

Policy documents from the UKCC, Department of Health and NHS Executive are having an impact on the future direction of education and training for nursing within the UK. *Fitness for Practice* (UKCC, 1999a), *Standards for Higher Level Practice* (UKCC, 1999b), *Agenda for Change* (NHSE, 1999) and

Making a Difference (DOH, 1999a) all promote the development of nursing competence and promote the implementation of a competence/outcomes-based approach to nurse education.

NHS Executive-funded projects have previously been commissioned that examined the relevance of national occupational standards to nursing (Storey *et al.*, 1995; O'Hanlon & Andrews, 1997); these concluded that such standards have much to offer the nursing profession, and suggested that national occupational standards provide a common language that can be used to describe nursing and articulate clearly expected performance. Competences also provide a potential national curriculum template that would assist education providers in devising curriculums and help to ensure that nurses completing programmes are 'fit for purpose' (O'Hanlon & Andrews, 1997). Consequently, professional bodies are increasingly aware of the need to deliver occupational competence (Conroy, 1996).

Previous research into professional competence has followed three main traditions:

(1) detailed specifications of competent behaviour in the tradition of behaviourist psychology combined with analytic techniques of observations of and consultations with, practitioners
(2) psychometric techniques to identify overarching qualities linked to excellent job performance, focusing on mid-career professionals and selection issues rather than training (this has been particularly influential in management training and development)
(3) cognitive constructs of competence that challenge the notion of equating what a person *can* do with what they are *observed* to do in a performance context. This has been argued by some to be the difference between competence (performance behaviour) and capability (behaviour in the workplace).

The issue of competence to practise is one that has been debated in nursing for a number of years. The main issues discussed in *Fitness for Practice*, *Fitness for Awards* and *Fitness for Purpose* (UKCC, 1999a, c, d) are particularly relevant to the preparation and development of nurses who work in secure environments. The key to 'fitness for purpose' and 'fitness for practice' lies in the ability of education commissioners and purchasers to reach agreement with the nurse education and training providers on the competence outcomes that a student should have acquired, and be able to use in practice, at the end of a nursing programme (Storey *et al.*, 1995).

A recent report on pre-registration training (UKCC, 1999a) provides the latest definition of competence directly related to nursing. It states that competence is 'the skills and ability to practice (*sic*) safely and effectively without the need for direct supervision'. Policy documents from the UKCC, Department of Health and NHS Executive are having an impact on the future direction of education and training for nursing within the UK. *Fitness for Practice* (UKCC, 1999a), *Standards for Higher Level Practice* (UKCC, 1999b), *Making a Difference* (DOH, 1999a), and *The Future Organisation of Prison Health Care* (DOH, 1999b) all promote the development of nursing competence and promote the implementation of a competence/outcomes-based approach.

Higher education institutions offer a wide range of specialist practitioner courses validated by the national boards for nursing and midwifery education. However, there does not appear to be a common understanding of competence to practise across education providers nor consensus on appropriate methods of assessing that competence (UKCC, 1997).

There are a significant number of definitions and types of competence described in the nursing and wider professional literature (WHO, 1988; Hogston, 1993; Mansfield & Mitchell, 1996; DOH, 1999a). From an analysis of this literature it can be ascertained that there are a number of forms of competence models (Mitchell, 1998), including:

- 'what people should be like' models based on personal characteristics or an individual's behaviour
- 'what people need to possess' models based on acquiring knowledge, understanding and skills
- 'what people need to achieve in the workplace' models based on outcomes and standards including underpinning knowledge and skills.

A two-stage process for deriving specific competences – 'job analysis' followed by 'skills analysis' – has been suggested. 'A job analysis is an investigation into the current job (what is?) and the future job (what ought to be).'

Skills analysis involves a consultative process between all stakeholders including maximum use of group processes involving employees who actually do the jobs (not just their supervisors). Other techniques of analysis may also be used, for example, general questionnaires and structured interviews.

The development of competences in the UK prison service

In delivering nursing and healthcare within a prison environment practitioners require competences that have evolved from a range of work areas. Prison healthcare not only includes meeting physical, mental health and learning disability needs of clients but must also be delivered in an environment that requires compliance with rigorous security policies and protocols.

In December 1999 a working party was established by Health Minister, Lord Hunt and Prisons Minister, Paul Boateng, to consider the development of nursing in prisons and the re-introduction of prison healthcare officers as members of a multi-disciplinary healthcare team. One of the key recommendations of the resulting report, *Nursing in Prisons* (DOH, 2000a) was 'that the Prison Service should commission a national occupational standards framework for prison nursing'. This approach reflects the trend that is emerging in relation to professional developments across nursing.

The competence definition described in *Nursing in Prisons* (DOH, 2000a) reflects these criteria. *Nursing in Prisons* defined competence as 'the knowledge, skill and attitude required for the performance of the occupational standards in a designated role or setting ...'. The competence must be:

- what is agreed is needed for the provision of good care
- demonstrated over time in practice in the real work setting
- assessed by a skilled and trained assessor.

A number of competence frameworks have been developed over the last few years or are currently being developed that have relevance to nurses working in the prison service. Most fit into the categories as defined by Mitchell (1998).

What people need to possess

In this category frameworks have been developed by the Registered Psychiatric Nurses Association of British Columbia and the Sainsbury Centre for Mental Health.

Registered Psychiatric Nurses Association of British Columbia

In a study in Canada, the Registered Psychiatric Nurses Association of British Columbia (Niskala, 1986, 1987) identified the following core competences:

- maintain security
- communicate effectively
- maintain records and prepare reports
- do counselling
- perform the nursing process

- plan and/or participate in programmes
- conduct and participate in groups
- perform and/or assist with diagnostic and treatment procedures
- maintain professional role
- carry out psychiatric nursing modalities
- participate in research projects
- instruct offenders, families and other staff
- perform administrative functions.

These standards were updated in 1998, and are now themed into seven main areas:

(1) provide competent professional care through the helping role
(2) perform/refine client assessments through the diagnostic and monitoring function
(3) administer and monitor therapeutic interventions
(4) effectively manage rapidly changing situations
(5) intervene through the teaching–coaching function
(6) monitor and ensure the quality of healthcare practices
(7) practise within organisational and work role structures.

These competences have some commonality with other frameworks, such as those developed by the Sainsbury Centre for Mental Health (1997, 2000), Watson and Kirby (1999), the University of Central Lancashire and Ashworth Hospital Authority (*Framework of Occupational Standards*, 1997 – unpublished), the standards in forensic social work (CCETSW, 1995) and the core competences for mental health workers commissioned by the NHS Executive North West Regional Office in 1998.

Sainsbury Centre for Mental Health

The Sainsbury Centre identified a number of core competences for mental health workers that have relevance for workers in secure settings. The twenty-nine core skills are divided into four main areas:

(1) management and administration
(2) assessment
(3) treatment and care management
(4) collaborative working.

These generic core skills are being subjected to further scrutiny and the Sainsbury Centre is currently reviewing these competences and consulting on the revised draft, which includes these key areas:

- social and practical interventions
- crisis interventions
- medical interventions
- psychological therapies
- continuing care and rehabilitation
- individual assessment and care planning
- carer support and intervention
- collaborative working
- lifelong learning.

What people need to achieve in the workplace

A number of models based on outcomes and standards including underpinning knowledge and skills are relevant to prison healthcare:

- State Hospital for Scotland security standards
- NMC pre-registration standards for progression to branch and entry to the register
- NMC higher level practice
- Custodial Care National Training Organisation standards
- Community Justice National Training Organisation standards
- Care NVQs
- University of Central Lancashire and Ashworth Hospital occupational standards.

State Hospital for Scotland security standards

The State Hospital at Carstairs has also developed competences for maintaining a safe environment. The competences are appropriate to all grades of nurses (Watson, 1999). The competences (occupational standards) were validated as S/NVQ units by SCOTVEC. The areas covered by the competences include:

- fire, searching, escorting, visitor control
- risk assessment/management
- assessment/management of dangerousness
- prevention/management of aggression

- observation, communication
- management of hostage and other security breaches.

Occupational standards have also been developed for delivering care and treatment including:

- anger management
- offence-related work
- reasoning and rehabilitation/moral reasoning and empathy
- social skills training
- psycho-education
- psychotherapies, counselling, psychosocial interventions.

(Watson, 1999)

NMC pre-registration standards for progression to branch and entry to the register

The UKCC/NMC pre-registration competences have been developed following the publication of *Fitness for Practice* (UKCC, 1999a), which identified the need to have outcomes for the end of year one, entry to the branch programme and for entry to the register.

Competences required for entry to the branch programme are:

- manage self, one's practice, and that of others, in accordance with the UKCC/NMC Code of Professional Conduct, recognising one's own abilities and limitations
- practise in accordance with an ethical and legal framework that ensures the primacy of patient/client interest and well-being and respects confidentiality
- practise in a fair and anti-discriminatory way, acknowledging the difference in beliefs and cultural practices of individuals or groups.

Competences required for entry to the register are:

- engage in, develop and disengage from therapeutic relationships through the use of appropriate communication and interpersonal skills
- create and utilise opportunities to promote the health and well-being of patients/clients and groups
- undertake and document a comprehensive, systematic and accurate nursing assessment of the physical, psychological, social and spiritual needs of patients/clients/communities

- formulate and document a plan of nursing care, where possible in partnership with patients/clients/carer(s)/significant others within a framework of informed consent
- based on best available evidence, apply knowledge and an appropriate repertoire of skills indicative of safe nursing practice
- provide a rationale for the nursing care delivered that takes account of social, cultural, spiritual, legal, political and economic influences
- evaluate and document the outcomes of nursing and other interventions
- demonstrate sound clinical judgement on a range of professional and care delivery contexts
- contribute to public protection by creating and maintaining a safe environment of care through the use of quality assurance and risk management strategies
- demonstrate knowledge of effective interprofessional working practices that respect and utilise the contributions of members of the health and social care team
- delegate duties to others, as appropriate, ensuring they are supervised and monitored
- demonstrate key skills in literacy, numeracy, application of information technology, problem-solving
- demonstrate a commitment to the need for continuing professional development and personal supervision activities in order to enhance knowledge, skills, values and attitudes needed for safe and effective nursing practice
- enhance the professional development and safe practice of others through peer support, leadership, supervision and teaching.

A number of universities are using these standards to adapt pre-registration programmes to enable students to be accredited with prior experience and learning. This may have potential benefits for the prison service as healthcare officers (HCOs) may be in a position to undertake a shortened course if they can demonstrate competence against these standards. In many instances, universities are using the care NVQ standards as a framework for inclusion on pre-registration programmes.

NMC *higher level practice*

The higher level of practice–pilot standard (HLP) also has relevance for the prison service as there are a number of practitioners within the service who fulfil the criteria because of the nature of their work.

The HLP standard encompasses the following areas of practice:

- providing effective healthcare
- improving quality and health outcomes
- evaluation and research
- leading and developing practice
- innovation and changing practice
- developing self and others
- working across professional and organisational boundaries.

Custodial Care NTO standards

The Custodial Care National Training Organisation (NTO) and the Community Justice NTO have developed a number of NVQs, which were introduced in 2002, for prison and community justice staff.

The key purpose of the custodial care standards is primarily to 'provide effective restrictions on people's liberty under the rule of law, treating them with care and humanity, in order to protect the wider community, reduce offending behaviour and help them to lead constructive lives' (Custodial Care NTO, 1999).

The six key areas are:

(1) strategy and policy: develop policies and strategies for effective custodial care and ensure their implementation
(2) management, administration and support services: maintain and develop the capacity of organisations and individuals to provide custodial care
(3) maintaining and developing work in custodial care: maintain and develop effective and safe working in custodial care
(4) security and restrictions on liberty: maintain security and restrictions on people's liberty under the rule of law
(5) needs and rights: meet people's individual needs and protect their human rights
(6) addressing offending behaviour: assist people to address their offending behaviour and lead more constructive lives.

The fifth key area, needs and rights, incorporates issues around inmates' health needs. There will be a number of units of competence specifically relating to healthcare, including the following:

- assess and review people's needs and rights
- plan, provide and modify programmes to meet people's needs and rights

- refer people to specialist services and support
- provide for people's dietary needs
- provide for people's hygiene needs
- provide for people's medical needs
- provide for people's childcare needs
- provide for people's physical exercise
- support people with difficult or potentially difficult relationships
- support people who are substance users
- support people who have been abused
- counsel people
- evaluate and deal with the potential to cause harm to self and others
- provide people with opportunities for outside contact
- provide people with opportunities for social contact within the custodial environment
- contribute to the protection of people within the custodial environment
- contribute to equal opportunities and human rights.

Community Justice NTO standards

The draft community justice standards include a number of areas of commonality as would be expected. These standards are provided for a multi-agency, multi-disciplinary team working outside custodial settings.

The six key areas are:

(1) develop, co-ordinate and maintain sector and agency effectiveness
(2) promote community safety, justice and social inclusion
(3) support individuals and families affected by crime
(4) manage the risk to the public of offending behaviour and develop programmes to address individuals' behaviour and related factors
(5) develop, implement and evaluate interventions to address behaviour, factors which contribute to it and risk
(6) foundations of all practice.

'Foundations of all practice' incorporates the following key roles:

- promote rights, responsibilities and diversity
- promote effective communication and relationships
- develop the knowledge and practice of individuals, teams and agencies
- build and sustain relationships between other workers and agencies.

These units appear in a number of frameworks, and are incorporated to a certain extent in the NMC pre-registration competences, the HLP standard and in the care NVQs.

Care NVQs

The units of competence that make up the care NVQs are wide-ranging and fairly comprehensive. Within the prison service the care NVQs have been used to develop the competence and acknowledge the skills of HCOs. A number of prisons across the country have worked with NVQ providers to develop an infrastructure of assessors and verifiers to support NVQ candidates for level 2 and level 3 NVQs in care.

University of Central Lancashire and Ashworth Hospital occupational standards

The University of Central Lancashire has worked with Ashworth Hospital Authority to develop a framework of occupational standards for staff working with patients with a severe personality disorder. These standards reflect the needs of staff and patients in a secure environment. Although they were specifically developed for the multi-disciplinary team working in a personality disorder unit, the standards are readily generalisable and transferable to other roles in nursing healthcare. These standards have been the subject of consultation, scrutiny and testing within the prison service across the UK. The results of the consultation are incorporated into the report *Nursing in Secure Environments* published by the UKCC in November 1999 (UKCC & University of Central Lancashire, 1999).

The secure environments project and the implications of its findings for the prison service

In attempting to identify the competences required of nurses working in a secure environment, the 'Job Competence Model' described by Mansfield and Matthews (1985) provided a framework for development. This model suggests that work roles have four interrelated components, all of which are present in all activity. The components are described as:

(1)   technical expectations: achieving the expectations of the work role which characterise the occupation
(2)   managing contingencies: recognising and resolving potential and actual

breakdowns in processes and procedures including coping with emergencies

(3)   managing different work activities: achieving balance and co-ordinating a number of different and potentially conflicting activities to lead to the successful conclusion of aims and goals

(4)   managing the interface with the work environment: achieving the expectations that arise from natural constraints, the quality measures that are applied, the nature of work organisation and the nature of working relationships.

In order to identify the competences that are required to work in secure environments a number of approaches were taken by the UKCC secure environments project team (UKCC & University of Central Lancashire, 1999). Individual interviews with managers, practitioners and educationalists were conducted, focus groups with practitioners from hospitals and the prison service were held, and questionnaires from employing organisations and individual nurses were distributed and analysed.

The questionnaire was distributed to a total sample of prison nurses and to a random sample of nursing staff in the secure health sector. Over 700 responses from registered nursing staff working in prisons or healthcare were received. (More than 328 responses were analysed from nurses in the England and Wales prison service.) The competences were clustered into groupings of similar interventions for analysis as to whether the respondent agreed that the competence was part of his or her role and the level of importance that the respondent attributed to the competence. When asked whether the competences were part of their role respondents replied either that:

- the competence was or was not part of their role; or
- they were responsible for supervising others in relation to the competence.

A significant number of staff indicated that specific competences were both part of their role and that they were responsible for supervising others in carrying out this task. From these data, a number of key themes emerged. These were primarily in relation to:

- safety and security
- assessment and observation, including risk assessment and management
- management of violence and aggression, control and restraint, de-escalation techniques

- therapies and treatments, including cognitive behaviour therapy (CBT) and psychosocial interventions (PSI)
- knowledge of offending behaviour and appropriate legislation
- report writing
- jail craft
- practical skills, including primary healthcare, first aid and practice nursing.

These themes reinforce findings from other studies (Niskala, 1987; Canadian Federation of Mental Health Nurses, 1998; Storey & Dale, 1998). In the field of nursing in secure environments, and particularly mental health, some work has been undertaken over the last few years by individual organisations and national bodies in order to identify the core competences that nurses require to provide effective nursing care to patients. The interventions can be clustered into five key areas as follows:

(1)   promote and implement principles that underpin effective, quality practice
(2)   assess, develop, implement, evaluate and improve programmes of care for individuals
(3)   develop, implement, evaluate and improve environments and relationships that promote therapeutic goals and limit risks
(4)   provide and improve resources and services that facilitate organisational functioning
(5)   develop the knowledge, competence and practice of self and others.
                                                                (Storey & Dale, 1998)

The responses indicate that there is a clear endorsement that the competences featuring in the UKCC study questionnaire are, in the main, part of the role and are rated as important or very important by the majority of nurses in both sectors. From the forty-five competences identified only five had a significant number of nurses from the prison services who said it was not part of their role, whereas hospital-based nurses viewed all of the competences as being part of their role.

The five competences with a low response rate in relation to being part of the prison nurse's role were:

(1)   promote the needs of individuals in the community
(2)   negotiate, agree and support placements for individuals
(3)   develop, monitor and review discharge packages to manage individuals
(4)   enable an individual's partners, relatives and friends to adjust to and manage the individual's loss

(5) enable individuals, their partners, relatives and friends to explore and manage change.

This response is not surprising as it reflects the current role and responsibilities of prison nurses. However, it is interesting to note that the Custodial Care NTO standards (DOH, 2000a) focus on a number of these areas.

One key finding of the analysis was the much higher reported level of both supervising and undertaking the role of supervisor in the health sector. This was consistent throughout the competences and was reported on average at over three times the level in health as in the criminal justice system. This finding may reflect the higher levels of skill/grade mix and numbers of nursing staff in the health sector as opposed to the prison nursing service. It does have implications for the number of staff who would be expected to develop supervisory skills and to pursue the dual role of both supervising and directly providing clinical care.

The competence framework adapted and evaluated during the UKCC *Nursing in Secure Environments* project (UKCC & University of Central Lancashire, 1999) has been validated by the 700 nurses who responded and provides an overarching framework from which further refinement can take place. This framework encapsulates occupational standards that have subsequently appeared in frameworks developed by other organisations. The NMC pre-registration and HLP standards can be clearly identified in this framework, as well as a number of standards from the Custodial Care NTO standards. The skills, knowledge and understanding identified in the Sainsbury Centre's core competences are also evident in the secure environments framework.

Conclusion and implications for the future

The UKCC identified that:

Competence based approaches to vocational and professional development have been increasingly advocated by UK governments and employers. Nurse education must reflect these needs. Higher Education institutions offer a wide range of National Board validated specialist practitioner courses but there does not appear to be a common understanding of competence to practise across providers nor consensus on appropriate methods of assessing that competence.

(UKCC, 1997)

The introduction of competence-based job descriptions enables employers and employees in the prison service to have a clear understanding of expectations in relation to role performance. This development also has impacts on training needs analysis and individual performance reviews, and provides a basis for developing validated, modular, continuing education packages. The identification and development of an integrated competence framework linked to health needs assessment would enable the prison service and other key stakeholders to identify the competences needed to meet the demands of the service and to use the framework when negotiating with education providers to develop education and training tailored to the needs of the service and staff. Classroom-based programmes do not need to be the main method of delivery; open and distance learning packages are available to support such a programme or can be developed.

The benefits of this type of approach are that modular programmes can be undertaken over a period of time and can therefore be more cost-effective for participants. They can be multi-disciplinary in nature, covering aspects of roles common to a range of healthcare professionals; or multi-sectoral, providing for the needs of both healthcare services and the prison service. They also allow progression that will enable participants to undertake appropriate modules and achieve accreditation for completed modules; and they have multiple entry and exit points, again meeting the needs of individuals and employers. This approach acknowledges previous experience and qualifications and, being flexible, it can be modified to meet changing needs.

Competences have a capacity to be utilised for assessing requirements and funding for national and local training provision and once implemented can be used to monitor the programmes' progress. The competences also provide coherence for the national provision of qualifications (including the development and updating of NVQs) and criteria for equivalence between national and international qualifications. At an individual level the development of the methods and processes of formal assessment systems based around competences can be a benchmark for assessing achievement. They also represent an ideal format for the collection of evidence for NVQs and a specification for summative assessment for other forms of public certification.

Allowing new learners to see the 'whole picture' in a simple and convenient format increases the relevance and credibility of the training/learning programme and enables learners to match the relevance of both the theory and the practice elements of training programmes. These programmes should not only address the skill/competence needs of the learners' organisations but also the learners' own individual learning needs. Arising from this is the use of a competences framework as a template for identifying previously acquired competence for individual action planning and identifying group learning needs. This can help with the development of a strategic view of future learning requirements and in the co-ordination of different human resource development processes. Also the competences can be usefully applied to specifying induction and initial training and in providing a transparency in learning outcomes and the development of learning contracts.

In summary, competences are a format for structured learning, help in identifying learning opportunities in the work environment and in broadening the scope and relevance of traditional skills-based training. They help to identify a progression route for learners by the development of knowledge content for learning programmes by way of specific learning objectives.

From an organisational perspective, competences can be utilised to link training to business objectives and assist in the evaluation and selection of learning resources against organisational requirements. If the training is to be provided externally to the organisation, as was the case in a large proportion of the forensic services responding in this study, the competences can be used as a specification of required outcomes and targets, for monitoring purposes, and in evaluating individual/group training programmes.

It is also important to consider how competences are necessarily assessed. Assessment is essentially both formative and summative; and incorporated into this is the creation of evidence for critical reflection. The assessment of skills and knowledge together involves a series of stages starting with the collection of evidence, which is reflected upon by the student, the mentor and the lecturer. There follows a need for dialogue between the student (who sees it as part of a discourse of learning), the mentor (who sees it as related to issues of practice and work), and the lecturer (who sees it as educational development). The dialogue allows separate interpretations to be discussed, learned from and integrated. It also builds in monitoring, in which assessment structures and mechanisms are evaluated in terms of how well they lead to the collection, analysis and critique of evidence.

This points to the processes of learning, assessment and professional activity. The implication is that the best means of developing and refining professional judgement, including assessments of competence, is through such a process. Nurses who are both 'knowledgeable doers' and 'reflective practitioners' are found most often where everyone involved in the programme of learning is engaged in a process of action, reflection, critique and further action (Philips *et al.*, 1993). The significance of this is that the learning essentially takes place in an applied way and is entirely relevant to the student's current clinical practice.

Competence-based models of development provide such a means for continuing professional development.

References

Canadian Federation of Mental Health Nurses (1998) *Competences for Psychiatric Nursing*. Registered Psychiatric Nurses Association of British Columbia, Vancouver.

CCETSW (1995) *Achieving Competence in Forensic Social Work*. Central Council for Education and Training in Social Work, London.

Conroy, M. (1996) *The Future Health Care Workforce*. Health Service Management Unit, Manchester University, Manchester.

Custodial Care NTO (1999) *Occupational Standards for Custodial Care*. Custodial Care National Training Organisation, Gateshead.

DOH (1998) *A First Class Service – Quality in the New NHS*. Department of Health, London.

DOH (1999a) *Making a Difference*. Department of Health, London.

DOH (1999b) *The Future Organisation of Prison Health Care*. Report by the Joint Prison Service and National Health Service Executive Working Group. Department of Health, London.

DOH (2000a) *Nursing in Prisons*. Report by the Joint Prison Service and National Health Service Executive Working Group. Department of Health, London.

DOH (2000b) *The Mental Health National Service Framework*. The Stationery Office, London.

Hogston, R. (1993) From competent novice to competent expert: a discussion of competence in the light of post registration and practice project (PREPP). *Nurse Education Today*, **13**(3), 341–4.

Mansfield, B. & Matthews, D. (1985) *The Components of Job Competence*. Further Education Staff College, Bristol.

Mansfield, B. & Mitchell, L. (1996) *Towards a Competent Workforce*. Gower Press, Oxford.

Mitchell, L. (1998) Paper presented at RCN Vocational Qualification Forum Conference, 10th May 1998, Liverpool.

Niskala, H. (1986) Competencies and skills required by nurses working in forensic areas. *Western Journal of Nursing Research*, **8**(4), 400–13.

Niskala, H. (1987) Conflicting convictions: nurses in forensic settings. *Psychiatric Nursing*, April, May, June, 10–14.

O'Hanlon, M. & Andrews, D. (1997) *Occupational Standards – A Framework for Clinical Effectiveness?* The Royal Liverpool University Hospitals, Liverpool.

Philips, M.S. (1983) Forensic psychiatric nurses: attitudes revealed. *Dimensions*, 60(9), 42–3.

Sainsbury Centre for Mental Health (1997) *Pulling Together: The Future Roles and Training of Mental Health Staff*. Sainsbury Centre for Mental Health, London.

Sainsbury Centre for Mental Health (2000) *Capability for Mental Health*. Sainsbury Centre for Mental Health, London.

Storey, L. & Dale, C. (1998) Nursing in Secure Environments. *Psychiatric Care*, 5(4), 214–18.

Storey, L., O'Kell, S. & Day, M. (1995) *Utilising Occupational Standards as a Complement to Nurse Education*. NHS Executive, Leeds.

UKCC (1997) *PREP – Specialist Practice: Consideration of Issues Relating to Embracing Nurse Practitioners and Clinical Nurse Specialists*. CC/97/46. United Kingdom Central Council for Nursing, Midwifery and Health Visiting, London.

UKCC (1999a) *Fitness for Practice*. United Kingdom Central Council for Nursing, Midwifery and Health Visiting, London.

UKCC (1999b) *Standards for Higher Level Practice*. United Kingdom Central Council for Nursing, Midwifery and Health Visiting, London.

UKCC (1999c) *Fitness for Awards*. United Kingdom Central Council for Nursing, Midwifery and Health Visiting, London.

UKCC (1999d) *Fitness for Purpose*. United Kingdom Central Council for Nursing, Midwifery and Health Visiting, London.

UKCC & University of Central Lancashire (1999) *Nursing in Secure Environments*. United Kingdom Central Council for Nursing, Midwifery and Health Visiting, London.

Watson, C. (1999) Caring for the mentally disordered offender: perspectives from Scotland. Paper delivered to RCN First National Conference in Forensic Healthcare, Belfast.

Watson, C. & Kirby, S. (1999) A two nation perspective on issues of practice and provision for professionals caring for mentally disordered offenders. In: *Forensic Nursing and Multi-disciplinary Care of the Mentally Disordered Offender* (D. Robinson & A. Kettles, eds.). Jessica Kingsley, London.

WHO (1988) *Learning to Work Together for Health*. Report of a WHO study group on multi-professional education for health personnel: a team approach. World Health Organization, Geneva.

Further reading

NBS (1995) *Competence to Practice*. A literature review on competence to practice. Nursing Board for Scotland, Edinburgh.

Robinson, D.K. & Kettles, A. (1998) The emerging profession of forensic nursing: myth or reality? *Psychiatric Care*, 5(6), 214–18.

Shuttleworth, M. (1993) *Articulating the Competence Movement and Professional Formation*. De Montfort University, Leicester.

- changes to nurse regulation
- negligence, the duty of care and the prison nurse
- confidentiality and consent
- the impact of the Human Rights Act 1998
- other legislation
- laws related to children and young people
- nursing in specialist environments such as a mother and baby unit and young offenders institutions.

Changes to nurse regulation

Nurses have been regulated under statute since 1919; midwives have been regulated since 1902. At the beginning of 2002 there were approximately 600 000 nurses, 90 000 midwives and 25 000 health visitors registered with the UKCC. Many nurses hold both midwifery and/or health visiting qualifications or other qualifications. The functions of the UKCC were:

- to establish and improve the standards of training of professional conduct for nurses, midwives and health visitors
- to determine the requirements for entry to training and the nature, content and standard of courses leading to registration
- to maintain a register of qualified nurses, midwives and health visitors who practise within the United Kingdom
- to deal with allegations of misconduct and fitness to practise owing to ill health or incompetence
- public protection.

The government's review of the Nurses, Midwives and Health Visitors Act 1997 is making changes to the regulation of the profession, and these will inevitably affect prison nurses. Three groups involving representatives and officials from England, Northern Ireland, Scotland and Wales were set up by the government to manage the changes. These were:

(1)   The legislative proposals group: they drafted the proposals for changes to the legislation and invited consultation.
(2)   The reference group: included representatives from key stakeholders from consumers, education, employers and various professions. They advised the legislative proposals group.
(3)   The change management group (CMG): there was an independent chair, supported by a project director. The first consultation document on the

future shape of the UKCC was published on 1 August 2000. A further statutory consultation document was published at the beginning of April 2001. This consultation period ended in June 2001 and the recommendations were considered by September 2001. The CMG managed the complex transition from the current arrangements to the new Nursing and Midwifery Council (NMC). A shadow Nursing and Midwifery Council was established during the transition period, and took over full responsibility at the beginning of April 2002.

While it is difficult to speculate on the overall changes and impact that the new regulatory body will have on prison nurses, it is clearly unlikely that there will be changes to principles enshrined in nurse regulation such as the following:

- The standards of clinical practice, education and the professional conduct of all nurses, midwives and health visitors should be clearly defined for nurses working in England, Ireland, Scotland and Wales.
- There must be systems in place to monitor the implementation and effectiveness of standards.
- Standard-setting and conduct procedures, including maintaining a register of all nurses, midwives and health visitors deemed fit to practise in the UK, should exist.

There will, however, continue to be changes within the regulation and administration of the profession as the NMC becomes more firmly established and continues to address the important issue of accountability.

Negligence, duty of care and the prison nurse

Negligence

Negligence has been defined in case law as:

> ... the omission to do something which a reasonable man, guided upon those considerations which ordinarily regulate the conduct of human affairs, would do ... or doing something which a prudent and reasonable man would not do.
>
> *Blyth* v. *Birmingham Waterworks Co Ltd* (1856 11 Ex 781)

More simply, this means a failure by a health professional to take 'reasonable care' when there is a duty on him/her to do so.

In relation to prison nurses, negligence comprises three elements:

man and had been negligent. As the police had been notified of the man's suicide attempts, this information should have been passed on to the prison authorities. The prison staff were not negligent in respect of the man's death. If the police had provided the necessary documents and information about the man's medical history, then the prison staff would have been alerted to the concerns and should have provided closer supervision by both prison officers and healthcare staff. This, in turn, might have prevented the man from taking his own life.

However, supposing the prison staff had received this information and could have anticipated what might happen to the prisoner. Then the staff would have owed a duty of care to the prisoner, to minimise the risk of his attempting suicide by observing him closely and ensuring that he was accommodated in a safe environment at all times. Had he then committed suicide, it is possible that prison staff might have been found negligent for failing to supervise the man closely.

Case example two Neil Ross Jamieson *v*. Royal Hospital Trust (1999)

A schizophrenic patient was admitted to an NHS hospital as an emergency and refused to stay against medical advice. He was registered as an outpatient in the NHS hospital and subsequently threw himself from the third floor of a car park and sustained injuries. The patient claimed that the hospital was negligent for failing to detain him under section 2 of the Mental Health Act 1983. The patient was awarded damages on the basis of 75% negligence on the grounds that he was still receiving treatment as an outpatient even though he had chosen not to receive inpatient care.

Standards of care

The basic test for negligence is whether a practitioner's conduct (in this case the prison nurse's) is reasonable, given all the circumstances of the case. Reasonable conduct would not be negligent, unreasonable conduct would be. Negligence means falling below the standard of the 'ordinary reasonable man' – who is often described as the 'man on the Clapham omnibus'. This means not doing something he or she ought to do, or omitting something which he or she should have done. The test is objective, based on the hypothetical person, and not subjective, based on the defendant. Liability hinges on how far the defendant has deviated from the 'reasonable' standard of care. The standard of the 'ordinary reasonable man' is not necessarily that of an average man. For example, the standard of an average motorist is expected to be very high, so would not be expected to fall even if a driver had not yet passed a driving test. Let me begin by offering some explanation of what constitutes a reasonable or a higher standard of care and breaches of duty of care by health professionals.

Breaches of duty of care

As a general rule, if a nurse acts in accordance with the common practice of other similar professionals, he or she is not negligent (*Roberge* v. *Bolduc* [1991] 78 DLR). However, a practice or procedure itself might be perceived as negligent. Where a person holds out him- or herself as having a specialist skill, for example, a Registered Mental Nurse (RMN) who has particular experience of working with emotionally disturbed patients, he or she will be judged by the objective standards of a reasonably competent RMN exercising that skill. (In *Maynard* v. *West Midlands Regional Health Authority* [1984] 1 WLR 634 it was held that 'a doctor who professes to exercise a special skill must exercise the ordinary skill of his speciality'.)

The *Bolam* test (*Bolam* v. *Friern Hospital Management Committee* [1957] 1WLR 582) is what a responsible body of peers would do in the circumstances, in this case, a prison nurse or a psychiatrist. The *Bolam* case suggested that a doctor was not negligent when acting 'in accordance with recognised medical practice, skilled and practised in that art' – in other words, the doctor has followed the practice of his or her profession.

The standard to be determined is the knowledge and practice that applied at the time of the alleged incident and not the time of the trial when practice and experiences may have changed (*Roe* v. *Minister of Health* [1954] 2 QB 66). The *Bolam* test has survived a number of legal challenges over the last few years. Now the *Bolam* test must be applied on the basis of both reasoned and considered assessment of the risks and benefits associated with the particular procedure in question (*Bolitho* v. *City and Hackney HA* [1998] AC 232). The *Bolam* test applies to nurses as well as to doctors.

Summary

- Negligence is caused by the failure to take reasonable care when there is a duty on the prison nurse to do so.
- The standard of reasonable care may vary with the expertise of the prison nurse.

There is generally no legal obligation to help victims of an accident outside the prison gates merely because those victims might benefit from assistance.

However, a district nurse or health visitor might be obliged by their contracts of employment to stop and care for an accident victim.

Human Rights Act 1998

The European Convention on Human Rights (ECHR) was a treaty of the Council of Europe signed in Rome in 1950. It aimed to protect Europe from a repeat of the genocide that occurred during World War II and to provide an unprecedented commitment to the protection of human rights. Many argue that its inception into UK law is long overdue. In Scotland the ECHR was introduced in 1999, since which time over 100 cases have been heard and 75 decided (RCN, 2001). In England and Wales, the Human Rights Act 1998 (the Act) came into force on 2 October 2000.

The provisions of the Act mirror many of those set out in the ECHR, and people can now claim their rights in UK courts and tribunals instead of having to apply to the European court in Strasbourg. The Act requires that public authorities, such as NHS organisations and the prison service, act compatibly with the ECHR. Over time, the Act will inevitably affect more issues in prison healthcare. The Articles of the ECHR that are given effect by the Act, and that have an impact on the prison nurse's work, include:

- the right to life
- prohibition against torture, inhuman or degrading treatment or punishment
- prohibition of slavery and forced labour
- the right to liberty and security
- the right to a fair trial
- no punishment without law
- the right to respect for private and family life
- freedom of thought, conscience and religion
- freedom of expression
- freedom of assembly and association
- the right to marry
- prohibition of discrimination
- restrictions on political activities of aliens
- limitations on use of restrictions on rights.

Some but not all of the Articles are discussed below. At the outset, it is important to establish that a matter may only be taken up in law by individuals who believe their rights have been infringed under the Act. Prison nurses could be asked to provide statements either in a professional capacity or as an expert witness because they deliver healthcare to prisoners.

Section 6 of the Act imposes a duty on public authorities to act compatibly with the European Convention on Human Rights, subject to specified exceptions. The Department of Health, health authorities, NHS trusts and prisons will be classified as 'obvious' public authorities under section 6.

Article 2 The right to life

The Articles that are likely to have impact on the duty of care are Article 2, the right to life, and Article 3, the prohibition on inhumane and degrading treatment. Both these Articles confer absolute rights.

The right to life has been acknowledged as 'the most fundamental of human rights' and calls for 'the most anxious scrutiny' (*Bugdaycay* v. *Secretary of State for the Home Department* [1987] AC 514 at 531G). The right to life was largely unexplored by UK domestic courts until the leading case of Tony Bland. This case concerned withdrawing life support treatment from a young person who was in a persistent vegetative state (PVS). Withdrawing treatment would result in death (*Airedale NHS Trust* v. *Bland* [1993] AC 789). The courts may in future be confronted with imaginative and progressive arguments as clients try to test the boundaries to the right to life.

In the case of *X* v. *UK* [1978] 14 D&R at 33, it was demonstrated that prison authorities must take 'adequate and appropriate steps to protect life' particularly when it has taken a person into custody (*X* v. *FRG Application No 10565/ 83* (1985) EHRR 152 at 153). Domestic courts may face the argument that health authorities and NHS trusts are obliged to make 'adequate and appropriate' provision for medical care in all those cases where a patient's right to life would otherwise be endangered. The right to life may also extend to cases where injury has occurred and it can be demonstrated there was a real and immediate risk to life (*Osman* v. *UK* [1999] 5 BHRC 293).

The courts will also give consideration to the duty imposed by Article 2 – the right to life – and the duty imposed by the domestic law of negligence. If an NHS trust is obliged to make adequate provision for medical care and fails to do so in circumstances where either death occurs or injury is sustained in circumstances where there was a real and immediate risk to life, a breach of Article 2 will have been established.

Article 3   No one shall be subjected to torture or degrading treatment or punishment

Although prisoners who are held on remand or serving a sentence of imprisonment lose their right to liberty, they may be offered some protection under Article 3. However, before Article 3 provisions can be considered, the prisoner must prove that he or she has been exposed to ill treatment that exceeds the threshold of Article 3. For example, IRA prisoners complained to prison officials about their detention in cells that they had personally smeared with food and faeces and that were uninhabitable and degrading (*McFreely* v. *United Kingdom* [1984] 38 D&R 11). While the European Commission (prior to the enforcement of the Human Rights Act 1998) recognised that the prisoners had self-imposed their conditions, it also recognised that the prison authorities have a responsibility for health and safety in prisons and should maintain cleanliness wherever possible in prison cells.

Prison authorities are obliged to ensure the health and well-being of all prisoners, within the prisoner's 'ordinary and reasonable requirements' (*McFreely and Others* v. *United Kingdom Applications 8317/8* [1980] 38 D&R 44 para 44). In exceptional cases, where a prisoner is too ill to receive specialist care in prison, the criminal justice system may be asked to consider humanitarian measures by transferring the patient to an outside hospital or hospice. In the case of Reggie Kray, who had a terminal illness in 2000, the Home Office permitted him to die outside the prison environment, close to his family and friends.

There is an obligation under Article 3 to provide medical treatment for persons detained in a mental hospital (*Hurtado* v. *Switzerland* [1994] Series A 280–A). The European Commission found that Article 3 had been violated, when a person who had been forcibly arrested was not given an X-ray until six days after he had requested it. The X-ray report revealed that the prisoner had a fractured rib.

Article 6   The right to a fair trial

Article 6 suggests that everyone has the right to a fair trial ('everyone' includes both the accused and those prosecuting). This also includes the right for all relevant evidence to be disclosed in the preparation of the trial (*Edwards* v. *United Kingdom* (1992) 15 EHRR 417). In criminal cases, the accused is presumed innocent until proved guilty 'beyond reasonable doubt' and is allowed certain rights in accessing legal advice, preparing and presenting a defence so that all the necessary arguments can be put before the court in a language that the defendant understands (Article 6(3)). Although there is no automatic right of appeal, under this Article, other articles may permit the defendant a right of appeal to a higher court (*Edwards* v. *United Kingdom* (1992) 15 EHRR 417 and Seventh Protocol: Article 2).

Article 8 The right to respect for private and family life

Everyone has the right to respect for their private and family life, their home and their correspondence.

In England, the prison estate includes mother and baby units, which may accommodate babies up to nine months of age in closed units or 18 months in open prisons. The recent case of *R (P)* v. *Secretary of State for the Home Department of the Divisional Court* (2001) held that it was lawful for the prison service to remove children from a mother's care when they reached the age of 18 months. In this case, a mother had contended that it was a breach of sections 1 and 17 of the Children Act 1989 (section 1: a child's needs are paramount; section 17 relates to a child in need) and Article 8 of the ECHR to remove her child. The court rejected the Children Act application and stated that Article 8(2) permits the state to interfere in family life in the interests of:

- public safety
- crime and disorder.

It also stated that the Home Office's decision to remove a child from his or her mother at 18 months was reasonable. The case does not appear to have addressed in detail the rehabilitation of the mother and the implications of separating the child from the mother at this stage.

An individual's medical records form an intimate part of his or her private life. Disclosure of such records, unless it can be justified with reference to Article 8(2) will constitute a breach of Article 8. (Examples where disclosure has been justified in the interests of public health include *TV* v. *Finland* [1994] 76-a-DR 140 Ecom HR; *Bolitho* v. *City and Hackney HA* [1998] AC 232; *Sidaway* v. *Governors of Bethlem Royal Hospital* [1985] AC 871; *Buckley* v. *UK* [1997] 23 EHRR CD 129). Disclosing the identity of someone with HIV and medical records that contain such information may not be relevant to a trial and could constitute a breach of Article 8 (*Z* v. *Finland* (1997) 25 EHRR 371). A recent case (*Edwards* v. *United Kingdom* (1992) 15 EHRR 417 and Seventh Protocol: Article 2) also raised issues about the rights of spouses not to give evidence against each other as well as breaches of confidentiality.

As yet, it seems that there is no duty on the prison authorities to provide conjugal rights for serving prisoners, thereby minimising an application being made under Article 12 – the right to found a family (*X and Y* v. *Switzerland* [1979] 13 D&R 242). However, it remains to be seen whether this may be challenged between prisoners and spouses and mental health patients or their partners.

Section 3 of the Sexual Offences (Amendment) Act 2000 concerns abuse of a position of trust, stating that:

... it shall be an offence for a person aged 18 or over

(a) to have sexual intercourse (whether vaginal or anal) with a person under that age; or
(b) to engage in any other sexual activity with or directed towards such a person,

if (in either case) he is in a position of trust in relation to that person.

(2) Where a person ('A') is charged with an offence under this section of having sexual intercourse with, or engaging in any other sexual activity with or directed towards, another person ('B'), it shall be a defence for A to prove that, at the time of the intercourse or activity

(a) he did not know, and could not reasonably have been expected to know, that B was under 18;
(b) he did not know, and could not reasonably have been expected to know, that B was a person in relation to whom he was in a position of trust; or
(c) he was lawfully married to B.

(3) It shall not be an offence under this section for a person ('A') to have sexual intercourse with, or engage in any other sexual activity with or directed towards, another person ('B') if immediately before the commencement of this Act

(a) A was in a position of trust in relation to B; and
(b) a sexual relationship existed between them.

(4) A person guilty of an offence under this section shall be liable

(a) on summary conviction, to imprisonment for a term not exceeding six months, or to a fine not exceeding the statutory maximum, or to both;
(b) on conviction on indictment, to imprisonment for a term not exceeding five years, or to a fine, or to both.

(5) In this section, 'sexual activity'

(a) does not include any activity which a reasonable person would regard as sexual only with knowledge of the intentions, motives or feelings of the parties; but

(b) subject to that, means any activity which such a person would regard as sexual in all the circumstances.

Meaning of 'position of trust'

4(1) For the purposes of section 3 above, a person aged 18 or over ('A') is in a position of trust in relation to a person under that age ('B') if any of the four conditions set out below, or any condition specified in an order made by the Secretary of State by statutory instrument, is fulfilled.

(2) The first condition is that A looks after persons under 18 who are detained in an institution by virtue of an order of a court or under an enactment, and B is so detained in that institution.

(3) The second condition is that A looks after persons under 18 who are resident in a home or other place in which

(a) accommodation and maintenance are provided by an authority under section 23(2) of the Children Act 1989 or Article 27(2) of the Children (Northern Ireland) Order 1995;

(b) accommodation is provided by a voluntary organisation under section 59(1) of that Act or Article 75(1) of that Order; or

(c) accommodation is provided by an authority under section 26(1) of the Children (Scotland) Act 1995,

and B is resident, and is so provided with accommodation and maintenance or accommodation, in that place.

(4) The third condition is that A looks after persons under 18 who are accommodated and cared for in an institution which is

(a) a hospital;

(b) a residential care home, nursing home, mental nursing home or private hospital;

(c) a community home, voluntary home, children's home or residential establishment; or

(d) a home provided under section 82(5) of the Children Act 1989,

and B is accommodated and cared for in that institution.

(5) The fourth condition is that A looks after persons under 18 who are receiving full-time education at an educational institution, and B is receiving such education at that institution.

(6) No order shall be made under subsection (1) above unless a draft of the order has been laid before and approved by a resolution of each House of Parliament.

(7) A person looks after persons under 18 for the purposes of this section if he is regularly involved in caring for, training, supervising or being in sole charge of such persons.

Article 12   The right to marry

Men and women of marriageable age have the right to marry and to found a family, according to the national laws governing the exercise of this right. Refusing a prisoner's right to marry might be seen as a violation of Article 12, although there is no requirement on the prison authorities to release the prisoner once married.

Article 14   Prohibition of discrimination

Article 14 states that the enjoyment of the rights and freedoms shall be secured without discrimination of sex, race, colour, language, religion, political or other opinion, national or social origin, association with a national minority, property, birth or other status.

Confidentiality

Principles of patient confidentiality

There are a number of statutory provisions that require information to be kept confidential. A legal obligation to preserve confidentiality is acknowledged in contract law and the duty of care in negligence.

Defining confidentiality

All paperwork, and now computerised material, generated in the course of employment is confidential. It is not there for any general member of the public to see. Those with a legitimate interest, for example, a supervisor, but not an inquisitive colleague, can see these documents/records in their professional capacity.

Specifically confidential information

Information conveyed with the specific request that it is to remain confidential should remain so. Confidentiality is usually implied by the nature of the communication and its sensitivity. Anything seen or heard in a professional capacity should be treated as such, but, for example, a conversation about the weather would not be confidential, whereas a comment about a prison governor's work visit to a conference with another colleague might be.

Permitted disclosure with consent

Essentially, a prison nurse should not break a confidence. However, there is no breach in the following circumstances:

- Express consent is given by the patient to share information with (an)other person(s) such as a senior member of staff. Sharing medical information may be limited. In other words, a male prisoner may be happy for a prison nurse to advise a prison medical officer about a medical condition, such as his anal warts. However, he has specifically asked the nurse not to inform any prison officers about this condition. As there would neither be a public interest nor arguably a specific 'need to know' basis about this particular condition, then the prison nurse should not inform any prison officer. To do so would constitute a breach of confidence on his or her part.
- Implied consent of the patient and/or client is given; that is, to other members of the healthcare team or relevant agencies on a need-to-know basis, and only such information as is necessary to achieve an objective, such as the best interests of a child who may be living either in or out of the prison.

Ownership of confidential information

Healthcare records are the property of your employer. There is no common law right of access to your records by the person who provided you with the information (*R* v. *Mid-Glamorgan Family Health Services and Another, ex parte Martin* [1993] PIQR 426).

Medical disclosure and confidentiality

Compulsory disclosure

NHS organisations have a common law duty of confidentiality. Personal information about patients held by health professionals is subject to a legal duty of confidence and should not be disclosed without the consent of the patient. Imparting any healthcare information without the consent of the patient/prisoner would generally be considered a breach of confidence.

Confidentiality should only be broken in exceptional circumstances and only after very careful consideration that such actions can be justified. The categories where a breach of confidence may be justified include giving evidence in court, statements made in the paramount interests of a child to legitimate inquirers, and in the public interest. The latter could apply to incidents that may occur in prison. The courts normally balance the public interests favouring confidentiality against those advising disclosure in the particular circumstances of each case. The question remains one for the courts and not for professional bodies (Kennedy & Grubb, 1998).

Prison nurses may be familiar with the leading case of *W* v. *Egdell* [1990] 2 WLR 471. This concerned W, who had been convicted of manslaughter after multiple killings in circumstances of extreme violence. He was detained under the Mental Health Act 1983 as a patient within a secure hospital. Dr Egdell was instructed by solicitors on behalf of W to prepare a psychiatric report. Dr Egdell believed that the contents of his report were of public interest as it contained information regarding W's dangerous behaviour and should be disclosed to the medical director caring for W and to the Home Office, to ensure that the public were not endangered by W's possible early release. The public interest of protecting the public from violence took precedence over the general public interest of ensuring the confidentiality of medical consultations.

Summary on confidentiality

- All health professionals are under an overriding ethical as well as a legal duty to protect the health and safety of their patients.
- The prison service should ensure that local procedures are in place relating to confidentiality and setting out the principles governing the appropriate

sharing of information, as per the *Health Service Circular HSC 2000/009: Data Protection Act 1998*.

In certain circumstances, it may be necessary to disclose or exchange personal information about an individual. This will need to be in accordance with the Data Protection Act 1998.

Data Protection Act 1998

The legal obligations imposed upon healthcare professionals who deal with confidential information supplied to them by patients are now largely codified by statute. The Data Protection Act 1998 implements the 1995 European Community Data Protection Directive. This regulates the use of personal information held on manual as well as computer records. The common law duty of confidentiality applies to personal data provided in confidence by patients. This must be complied with to meet the first principle of the Data Protection Act 1998, which requires fair and lawful processing of information.

The Data Protection Act 1998 does not itself prevent NHS bodies from using personal data for legitimate medical purposes, which may include the management of healthcare services (the Data Protection (Subject Access Modification) (Health) Order 2000 published on 23 March 2000). The *Health Service Circular HSC 2000/009: Data Protection Act 1998: Protection and Use of Patient Information* (published 23 March 2000) highlights the main implications for the NHS of the Data Protection Act 1998, associated Orders and Regulations and the actions NHS trusts must take in order to comply with the new legislation.

Summary

- All staff dealing with personal information must comply with the Data Protection Act 1998 and associated provisions, in particular those concerning the rights of data subjects (patients) in respect of access to and use of information in their health records.
- All staff dealing with personal information must be aware of the requirements of the common law duty of confidentiality. Any negotiations with a third party to process personal data on behalf of the organisation must be the subject of a written contract, which must comply with appropriate security and confidentiality arrangements.

Young offenders institutions (YOI)

A young offenders institution (YOI) is a place for offenders sentenced to detention in such institutions (Prison Act 1952, section 43(1)(aa)). According to Home Office statistics, in 2000 there were 8,046 young offenders aged 15–21 in prison, 7,697 male and 349 female. There are different definitions of a young person. The most common are as follows:

- A person who has attained the age of 14 years but who is under 17 years (Children and Young Persons Act 1933, section 107(1)).
- However, a child is a person under the age of 18 (Children Act 1989, section 105(1), subject to paragraph 16 of schedule 1).
- Prior to the James Bulger case, it was presumed that no child under the age of 10 years can be guilty of any offence (Children and Young Persons Act 1933, section 50).

The local authority must provide for the reception and accommodation of children removed or kept away from home:

- under Part V of the Children Act 1989, section 21
- where a child has been removed into police protection and the authority is requested to provide accommodation (Children Act 1989, section 46(3)(f))
- where an arrested juvenile has been kept in police detention and the arrangements are made for him to be accommodated (Police and Criminal Evidence Act 1984, section 38(6), as substituted by schedule 12, paragraph 26).

Young offenders

Some defendants accused of committing serious crimes may be very young and very immature when standing trial in the Crown Court. The purpose of such a trial is to determine guilt (if this is an issue) and decide the appropriate sentence if the young defendant pleads guilty or is convicted. The trial process should avoid exposing the young defendant to avoidable intimidation, humiliation or distress. All possible steps should be taken to assist the young defendant to understand and participate in the proceedings and to meet those ends. Regard should be had to the welfare of the young defendant (as required by the Children and Young Persons Act 1933, section 44).

Secure accommodation

This is accommodation provided for the purpose of restricting liberty (Children

Act 1989, section 25(1)). Such accommodation is generally used for young people who have a history of absconding from, for example, residential care and are likely to abscond from other accommodation and suffer significant harm or cause harm to others. These differ from secure detention centres.

Secure accommodation units in England and Wales (up to 31 March 1998)

In March 1998 there were 456 approved places in secure units, 436 in England and 20 in Wales. There has been a 33% increase in provision of places in England since March 1997 as a result of the secure accommodation programme.

Mothers and babies in prison

In 2001 there were four mother and baby units in HMP service in England:

(1) Holloway Prison, London: closed unit
(2) Styal prison, Manchester: closed unit
(3) Askham Grange, York: open prison
(4) Wakefield Prison: closed unit.

The Children Act 1989 aimed to give greater rights to the child and remove the distinction from public and private law. The child's rights under the Children Act 1989 are fundamental – but were not always considered before this piece of legislation. Prior to the Children Act 1989, a baby in prison was accommodated there by virtue of the mother's custodial and/or remand sentence.

The House of Commons Select Committee of Inquiry 1985 aimed to:

- recognise the needs of children accommodated in a prison setting
- provide, where possible, developmental screening/assessments by health visitors and medical staff for babies out of the prison setting
- ensure that no mother is manacled to a prison officer during labour
- ensure that mothers and babies have the choice to see a medical specialist, if indicated, outside the prison setting
- ensure that all births take place in hospital, out of prison
- ensure that a contract of care is discussed and agreed by the mother with prison staff for all mothers wishing to keep their babies in prison
- provide more nursery nurses after the initial postnatal period, to give support and advice regarding child development and infant nutrition

- improve accommodation and the layout for mothers who keep their babies with them in prison.

During the course of the inquiry, health visitors and medical staff made the following points:

- There should be better systems in place to address 'bonding' and separation of babies from their natural mothers.
- There is a need to consider early separation for women who have potentially long sentences, in order to minimise any emotional harm that might be caused by delaying separation.
- There is a need for appropriately trained 'volunteer' nurses and officers to work on the mother and baby unit. Neither nurses nor officers should be obliged to work on a mother and baby unit against their wills.
- It is important to organise a period of 'home leave' for those mothers with a baby in advance of the mother completing her sentence, to ensure that both are prepared for their return to the community.

The introduction of the Prison Service Mother and Baby Admission Boards in 2000 aimed to ensure that mothers who are accommodated with their babies in prison are vetted appropriately. This is to ensure that the child's best interests are at all times considered before being received into a prison environment.

Conclusion

Norman and Parrish (2001) recognise that 'nurses will always have a role to play in empowering their patients to have more control over their lives, particularly in the area of their health needs ... and have a special relationship with their patients'.

While the last two decades have seen an increase in the number of new laws, regulations and case law, which recognise and have challenged the duties owed by nurses to patients, increased public awareness of some of the rights to which prisoners may now be entitled suggests that the challenges for nurses working in a prison setting have never been greater.

However, such challenges should not be viewed with suspicion but seen rather as positive measures to bring about change. Prison nursing should be acclaimed as a worthwhile speciality that responds to the needs of society's most vulnerable and needy members. Both the staff who work in prisons and those held on remand or serving sentences in such environments must be supported and protected by healthcare policies and laws that are appropriate to this millennium.

References

Gannon, S. (2001) HiMSP, LIT and Thr'Penny bits: reception. *The RCN Newsletter for Prison Nurses*, 1.

JM Consulting Ltd (1998) *The Regulation of Nurses, Midwives and Health Visitors*. Report on the review of the Nurses, Midwives and Health Visitors Act 1997, JM Consulting Ltd, London.

Kennedy, I. & Grubb, A. (1998) *The Principles of Medical Law: Confidentiality and Medical Records*, para. 9.29, p. 503.

Norman, A. & Parrish, A. (2001) Volunteers in prison should be encouraged. *British Journal of Nursing*, **10**(1), 5.

RCN (2001) How the new Human Rights Act affects nurses. *Issues in Nursing*. Royal College of Nursing, London.

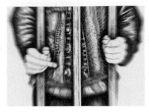

8 Quality Healthcare
Inspectorate Issues

MAGGI LYNE

The prison inspectorate team's aim is to raise the operational standards of establishments being inspected. This is achieved by a mixture of planned, announced inspections, each lasting a week, and short unannounced inspections, designed to examine a particular aspect or problem, to follow up a previous inspection, or to ensure that no prison goes for too long without some form of inspection. It is a unique role that gives the inspectorate an insight into the wider workings of the prison service. This chapter considers the views of a past member of Her Majesty's Prison Inspectorate team.

'Where imprisonment is imposed, loss of freedom constitutes the punishment, the health and well being of prisoners must not be compromised.'

(WHO, 1998)

Background

During the 1990s considerable publicity was given to the low standards of healthcare experienced by prisoners in England and Wales. Low standards of care, such as poor primary care, poor mental healthcare and the professional isolation of staff, found during inspections by Her Majesty's Inspectorate of Prisons (HMIP), were criticised in several inspection reports. These conditions led to HM Chief Inspector of Prisons publishing a discussion document *Patient or Prisoner?* (HMIP, 1996) in November 1996 in which the Chief Inspector recommended a two-year debate on when the NHS should assume responsibility for prisoners' healthcare.

A joint working group of officials from the prison service and the NHS

Executive was established by the Home Secretary and the Secretary of State for Health to consider 'the future organisation of, and ways of improving prisoners' health care'. The working group's report *The Future Organisation of Prison Health Care* (DOH, 1999) was published in March 1999. The report endorsed the aim for prison healthcare 'to give prisoners access to the same quality and range of health care services as the general public receives from the National Health Service'. It recommended a formal partnership between the prison service and the NHS including a substantial programme of change to remedy the weaknesses found.

The recommendation of the working group – a formal prison service–NHS partnership, rather than full transfer of responsibility for prison health, including funding, to the NHS – is welcomed as a big step forward in the short term. However, in the longer term, the NHS should take over full operational responsibility for prison healthcare. There will always be a need for partnership working at all levels in the service, but responsibility for improving healthcare in our prisons must be vested in the NHS locally, because healthcare in prison is inextricably bound up with healthcare in the community from which all prisoners come and to which the vast majority will return.

Key levers of change

Responsibility is placed on prison governors and health authorities, first, to identify the health needs of prisoners and, second, to prepare a prison health improvement strategy for each prison. This will form an intrinsic part of the wider health improvement programme being developed by health authorities for their populations in partnership with local authorities and other agencies. Health improvement programmes led by health authorities, embracing the whole population as they do, need to be grasped as the main engine of change to improve the health of the community in a way that includes everyone. At last, prisoners' health and its improvement is set fair and square in a formal partnership between prison governors and health authorities having joint responsibility for:

- identifying the health needs of prisoners
- agreeing a local prison health improvement strategy
- planning and commissioning the provision of needs-based prison healthcare, aiming for seamless provision by the prison and the community
- monitoring the progress of each health improvement strategy against a background of performance management.

Progress with caution

It is possible that the language of health improvement strategies and health improvement work programmes and so on can be a real switch-off for staff in prison healthcare, working as they do in close daily contact with prisoners and with all the demands placed on them. A reaction of 'So what? – a paper exercise of no relevance!' is likely and understandable, given the day-to-day pressures of working in such a very different and complex environment. Those who may feel sceptical about actual improvement happening on the ground can take comfort from the fact that at least mechanisms have been put in place to facilitate the necessary improvements. For the first time, new formal responsibilities, as outlined earlier, have been placed on governors and health authorities in relation to prison healthcare, and a Prison Health Policy Unit and Task Force have been set up centrally and charged with improving the quality of healthcare for prisoners. Never let it be said that just because structures have been put in place improvements will happen. However, in this instance, because of the government's focus on partnership working and improving quality of healthcare throughout the whole country, the Prison Health Policy Unit and Task Force will be working within a national culture of getting things done and making sure that patients notice real improvements in their treatment and care. The quality vision alongside the health improvement work programme prepared by the Policy Unit and Task Force during the summer of 2000 to implement required improvements should be known to all healthcare staff working in prisons.

Structural changes

The setting up of the Prison Health Policy Unit and Task Force creates accountable forums to provide leadership in remedying deficiencies in prison healthcare and in spreading news of good practice. The heads of the Policy Unit and the Task Force are accountable jointly to the Chief Executive of the NHS and the Director-General of the prison service. It is exceedingly important that the communication loop from the Policy Unit and Task Force embraces and engages governors and clinical staff in an orderly programme of change over the years ahead. This means that the changes must be known to governors and staff on the ground in prisons as well as to staff in the NHS. The heads of the Policy Unit and Task Force should be out and about in prisons learning about the actual improvements needed and supporting staff as changes and improvements are made. It is also important that staff believe that they have champions at the most senior level in the service who are dedicated to improving prison healthcare. It would probably be useful for a hotline or confidential helpline to be available in the Task Force office for prison healthcare staff to report areas of concern when local resolution fails.

At the start of this new century, we have cause to celebrate the initiatives taken, particularly because responsibilities have been given to named individuals to make real improvements in prison healthcare, who can be called to account at the highest level. Only time will tell what will be achieved. By 2003, the improvements in the quality of prison healthcare should be evident throughout the country. I, personally, am very hopeful provided that the formal partnership arrangements between the NHS and the prison service, as constructed in the Policy Unit and Task Force at national level, are reflected in relationships throughout the service at all levels with healthcare staff in prisons feeling empowered, liberated and resourced to do the very best they can for patients in their care, freed at last to be the professionals they are trained to be.

Options for nursing

The new climate of formal partnership between the prison service and the NHS creates opportunities for prison nurses to take the initiative individually and collectively, as champions of good healthcare for prisoners, to make real and practical improvements in the everyday lives of patients and themselves. Nurses will then be able to say, 'I can make a difference'. Prison nurses in partnership with their clinical colleagues in each prison should contribute to the preparation of the health improvement strategy and work programme so that there is ownership throughout the service and commitment to the changes ahead through real local involvement.

A singular omission in the joint prison service–NHS working group's recommendations and action points (DOH, 1999) was the absence of any meaningful reference to consulting prisoners about their health needs or listening to their views and opinions about the quality of the healthcare they receive. The prisoner's voice was silent in the report and ways must be found to enable prisoners' voices to be heard.

Seeking views

Over the years, having listened to patients individually and in groups during inspections, it has often been mentioned that nobody asks patients what they think or listens to what they have to say. Most comments are open and frank within this working relationship, which guarantees anonymity, and this makes prisoners feel safe to reveal their opinions. All in all, when a follow-up check is done, we find that prisoners have been honest with us. In fact, patients' opinions give a special focus to inspections and very often patients have underestimated the gravity of situations. So many times patients have said, 'I am a prisoner after all Miss, I can't expect much, can I'.

Prison nurses should build their advocacy role by helping and encouraging prisoners to speak for themselves and speaking up for those who cannot. No programme of improvements in prison healthcare would make sense without the views of patients being sought. It is a matter of respect for the individual. The patient knows best and nurses should insist that the patient's experience of the quality of healthcare provided is at the very heart of any changes and priorities for improvements in service delivery. It is also a matter of rights. Prisoners, though deprived of their liberty by the courts, retain their other rights including their right to healthcare equivalent to that provided to the rest of the community. The government now places great emphasis on listening to patients' views and consulting them on arrangements for their care in the wider NHS – prisoners should be consulted in exactly the same way about their health needs. No person should be worse off in terms of his or her healthcare because of being a prisoner.

The influence of nurses

Nurses are pivotal to health improvement programmes. It is a matter of common sense: as there are more nurses than other clinical staff, it follows that nurses spend more time with patients. They are thereby offered rich opportunities to help patients to improve their health, provided nurses are properly trained and suitably skilled. Nurses should examine ways to increase their personal clinical skills to match patients' needs and to avoid professional isolation through clinical supervision and by maintaining strong links with the NHS locally.

The success of the new formal partnership between the prison service and health authorities is contingent on changes taking place to improve the quality of care in each prison. It is the healthcare practitioners who will have the greatest influence in improving quality through daily contact with patients, in providing intelligence on what needs to change, in not tolerating poor standards and in working positively with the NHS, the Task Force and the Policy Unit to build better healthcare in prisons. For this reason, it is vital that all clinical staff throughout the prison healthcare service are involved in creating the changes to come and that they know and fully understand the reasons for priorities or pilots outlined in the health improvement strategy work programme.

A number of questions emerge for nurses from the publication of the report on *The Future Organisation of Prison Health Care* (DOH, 1999). The main one is whether nurses working in prison know about things that are happening centrally and locally to improve prisoners' healthcare as a consequence of the report's publication. How involved are prison nurses in responding to the report and influencing the changes? Do prison nurses know and understand the health improvement strategy for their prison and their own contribution to achieving the objectives set? Were prisoners' views sought in the preparation of the health improvement strategy? Do prison nurses know and understand the national quality vision designed to improve the quality of prison healthcare and the work programme, which supports the vision, and how has the vision been interpreted and understood locally?

The UKCC

The United Kingdom Central Council for Nursing, Midwifery and Health Visiting Code of Professional Conduct (UKCC, 1992) (to be replaced in June 2002 with an updated NMC code) requires that each nurse

> ... shall act at all times in such a matter as to:
> * safeguard and promote the interests of individual patients and clients; serve the interests of society; justify public trust and confidence, and uphold and enhance the good standing and reputation of the profession.

To fulfil these obligations, nurses must keep themselves up to date professionally and abide by 16 other requirements of the code.

Although all the 16 requirements of the *Code of Professional Conduct* (UKCC, 1992) apply to nurses, midwives and health visitors working in prison in the same way as the code applies to those nurses working outside prison throughout the United Kingdom, six of the requirements are of particular relevance for nurses working in the complexity of a prison healthcare environment (UKCC Codes 2, 7, 8, 10, 11, 12).

Nurses have to 'ensure that no action or omission on their part or within their sphere of responsibility, is detrimental to the interests, condition or safety of patients'. The word 'omission' here is significant as it emphasises that not doing something that ought to be done in the patient's interest can be as detrimental to the patient as doing something wrong. Here, I would include as examples of sins of omission: not assessing patients properly; not supporting the weak and frail in mind or limb; not making sure that patients get the care they need when it is readily available; not giving direct care to patients, with nurses using the prison environment as the excuse for no direct patient contact; allowing social isolation and occupational deprivation; tolerating poor standards and doing nothing about them. The question I often ask is, 'How can nurses working in prison leave mentally ill patients and other patients locked up for 22 hours a day and do nothing about it?' It does happen. I have seen it frequently.

Nurses have to 'recognise and respect the uniqueness and dignity of each patient and client, and respond to their need for care, irrespective of their ethnic origin, religious beliefs, personal attributes, the nature of their health problems or any other factor' (UKCC, 1992). 'Any other factor' is an inclusive phrase implying, as it does, any other personal situation a patient may be in such as imprisonment. The nurse's duty is constant and consistent, honouring the individual, and providing care to meet each patient's unique health needs in a variety of environments. Nurses need to know and understand the problems, complexity and limitations of the environment of care in which they work and they should be properly trained to practise safely in that environment. The prison healthcare environment presents particular problems and risks that may complicate nurses' ability to respond to prisoners' need for care in the same way as they would in, say, a GP practice outside prison, because the environments of care are completely different. The key problem for prison nurses is commonly called the caring/custody conflict; tensions can occur between caring and custodial duties and priorities for nurses practising in a prison environment. There is an urgent need for the interface between custody and caring to be examined by the NMC and for clear guidance to be issued on any special circumstances that a prison nurse may experience, and the risks that the nurse may encounter, owing to the nature of the environment of care. The confidence of the prisoner in the patient–nurse relationship and in the professional integrity and duty of the nurse should never be compromised. Recognition must be given to situations and environments that may compromise the nurse's ability to provide spontaneous, direct care to patients. The NMC has to face the professional challenges and occupational hazards presented to nurses by the prison environment and clarify those areas where professional conflicts are emerging.

Prison nurses should read their code of professional conduct regularly. The code alerts nurses to good and bad practice; it provides a checklist for reflection and examination of standards of practice and also gives nurses the leverage to do something about poor standards. It is well worthwhile examining each statement in the code to discern and recognise areas of difference or complexity inherent in the prison healthcare environment so that the environment of care is not jeopardised or damaged by false assumptions and restrictive practices.

Nurses have to 'protect all confidential information concerning patients and clients obtained in the course of professional practice and make disclosures only with consent, where required by the order of a court or where [the nurse] can justify disclosure in the wider public interest'. A number of questions arise here regarding patient confidentiality in prisons. Who has the right of access to patients' records in prison? Who supervises and authorises that access? Can the patient exercise his or her right of access to personal records? Are clinics/sick parades organised in such a way as to ensure patient confidentiality? Consultations have been seen taking place through door hatches with a queue of patients listening to the patient ahead, thereby compromising the patient's opportunity to confide. Confidentiality and identification of patients are two areas for quality improvement in prisons if each patient is to be respected and be safe. These issues are discussed in more detail in Chapter 7.

The UKCC/NMC code requires nurses 'to report to an appropriate person or authority regarding circumstances and conditions in which patient care may be adversely affected' in the following four instances:

(1)   at the earliest possible time, any conscientious objection which may be relevant to professional practice
(2)   any circumstances in the environment of care, which could jeopardise standards of practice
(3)   any circumstances in which safe and appropriate care for patients and client cannot be provided and
(4)   where it appears that the health and safety of colleagues is at risk, as such circumstances may compromise standards of practice or care.

My purpose in discussing the UKCC/NMC code of professional conduct for nurses is to emphasise the rights of prisoners to receive nursing care equivalent to that available on the NHS and to demonstrate that those working in prison have no licence to treat a prisoner with less respect than he or she would receive in the NHS out of prison. Working in prison presents special challenges in its complexity and environment; nonetheless, the problem areas must be openly explored and resolved to enable nurses to work safely to professional standards.

Needs of prisoners

Prisoners, by virtue of their loss of liberty, are the walled-off members of society and need protection to ensure that they are treated decently and humanely. Because of being hidden away from the rest of the community, prisoners' rights are easily infringed, and it could be argued, where healthcare is concerned, that the duty of the nurse is of a higher order owing to the nature of the risk presented to the patient by the closed environment. There are boards of visitors in each prison to monitor conditions and HMIP to provide independent inspection of the treatment of and conditions for prisoners. The chaplaincy teams have a significant role in supporting prisoners. Staff from several external organisations work in prisons, such as teachers, drug workers, volunteers, nurses, medical staff, etc. All these people are sources of refreshment in the prison culture.

During the 1990s, there was a substantial increase in the numbers of nurses employed in prison healthcare. The quality of healthcare provided to prisoners improved in some prisons but not in others. More than 20 new nurses were appointed to a prison, all new to prison life. None was given the essential training to introduce them confidently to working in prison healthcare. Several left within months. Those who remained were drawn unquestioningly into the discipline culture, with negative consequences for prisoners' healthcare.

The introduction of civilian nurses into prison healthcare, now known as prison nurses, was badly managed, and many nurses were casualties of the lack of induction or training in nursing in prison environments. The training of prison nurses and healthcare officers has been examined by a working party, whose report was published in 1999 (DOH, 1999). The professional isolation of clinical staff in prison must cease and plans to achieve this should form part of clinical governance quality assurance.

Professional responsibilities

The duty of the nurse and the nurse–patient relationship are set out clearly in the 1992 *UKCC Code of Professional Conduct* and other supporting UKCC documents. In some prisons HMIP has found appalling conditions in healthcare. It seemed as if nurses had surrendered their code of professional conduct on entering the prison gates. Of course, there were others in the prison with responsibility too: doctors, managers, the governor and so on, but here we are talking about nurses and the personal and professional accountability of the nurse. The most recent inspection prior to the writing of this chapter was in the spring of 2000.

In many instances, nurses felt disempowered and disabled by the prison culture and by the management in prison healthcare. During inspections, nurses have spoken to me as individuals and in groups; they knew only too well the deficiencies in the service provided, but felt they had little voice or influence. In the early and mid 1990s in particular, the caring versus custody conflict or divide was chiasmic and the nurses lacked any means or forum for discussing and resolving the problems. It is a tribute to so many prison nurses that they remained working in prison healthcare, seeking to improve the lot of prisoners, in spite of the limitations surrounding them. Many felt that their skills were not used to the full.

General management was introduced to the NHS during the 1980s, following the publication of the Griffiths report in October 1983 (DOH, 1983). Prison healthcare did not follow suit. During the course of our inspections, we observed confusion and overlap between the roles of senior medical officers and the governor grade in charge of healthcare. Responsibility and accountability demarcation lines were unclear. In most cases, there was no single person holding personal responsibility for the general management of healthcare. This was also the case in the NHS until the Griffiths team reported in 1983. The Griffiths report noted: 'Absence of general management support means that there is no driving force seeking and accepting direct personal responsibility for developing management plans, and securing their implementation, and monitoring actual achievement'. In his *Annual Report of HM Chief Inspector of Prisons for England and Wales 1997–98* (HMIP, 1998) the Chief Inspector of Prisons recommended that 'a new role of general manager in prison healthcare should be created and selection for the post holder should be based on a management track record of achievement, the primary profession being irrelevant'. Staff in prison healthcare 'have to be assured that when changes are being made, demands made on them will, as far as possible, be part of an orderly process'. With the amount of change facing prison healthcare, the first priority and action of the Prison Health Task Force and governors has to be the appointment of a healthcare manager for each prison with full general management responsibility which is defined as leading, planning, implementing, controlling and monitoring the total performance of the healthcare service for prisoners. Without this first essential step, and without the postholder being directly accountable to the governor, the management of the vital changes ahead will be flawed from the outset.

The NHS plan

The New NHS: Modern – Dependable (DOH, 1997) states:

> The new NHS will have quality at its heart. Without it, there is unfairness. Every patient who is treated in the NHS wants to know that they can rely on receiving high quality care when they need it. Every part of the NHS and every one who works in it, should take responsibility to improve quality.

A First Class Service – Quality in the New NHS (DOH, 1998) sets out how quality care, as a right for every patient, will be assured through a system of clinical governance and states that 'the drive to place quality at the heart of the NHS is not about ticking checklists – it is about changing thinking'.

Clinical governance is defined as 'a framework through which NHS organisations are accountable for continuously improving the quality of their services and safeguarding high standards of care by creating an environment in which excellence in clinical care will flourish'. The importance of clinical governance is that it 'provides NHS organisations [including prison healthcare] and individual health professionals with a framework within which to built a single, coherent local programme for quality improvement'. This means a multi-disciplinary approach to quality, and 'performance will be monitored by the NHS Executive' with 'independent scrutiny being provided by the Commission for Health Improvement'.

The government has set quality as the 'top priority for all NHS Trusts', requiring trusts 'to ensure proper processes are in place for assuring and improving quality, that they nominate a single person to lead the development of clinical governance and publish annual reports on action and progress. The named clinician can be a senior consultant, a nurse or other health professional'. For additional information on clinical governance and on the role of the National Institute of Clinical Excellence and the Commission for Health Improvement, prison nurses should read *A First Class Service – Quality in the New NHS* (DOH, 1998) and obtain a copy of their local clinical governance framework.

The government's drive for an improved health service, giving top priority to quality, has to be the opportunity and inspiration that healthcare staff in prison need. Because now there are obligations that empower prison healthcare staff of all specialities and grades to raise standards and refuse to have sub-standards as the norm where they exist. In addition, clinical governance 'provides the framework for a more coherent approach to local

Continuing Professional Development – life-long learning – which will, in turn, support improvements in service quality' (DOH, 1998). This means that there is now a direct relationship between the knowledge and skills of healthcare staff and the needs of patients for those skills. Each prison needs to have a champion for quality improvement through clinical governance. Could that be you?

It is important that the clinician, designated as responsible for ensuring that systems for clinical governance are in place in each prison, has the confidence of all clinical staff. A number of nurses have spoken to me about access to the governor on clinical and other matters. The lead clinician will probably chair a clinical governance multi-disciplinary group or committee, which will have nursing representation, and this is the forum for the quality of the service to be debated. Prisoners should have the quality of their healthcare ensured through clinical governance in a manner equivalent to that provided for patients in the NHS. Ideally, clinical governance for prison healthcare should form part of local NHS clinical governance arrangements.

Because only bad inspection reports get extensive press coverage, the impression is given that all prison healthcare is as bad as the worst publicity. But this is not the case. There are models of good practice across the service and a tremendous commitment by governors and clinical staff to improving the quality of healthcare in prison. The good news is that mechanisms are now in place to promulgate good practice and to raise standards generally, bringing poor performers up to the standards of the best through professional groups identifying remedies as part of clinical governance.

Despite improvements in prison healthcare and examples of good practice throughout the service, there is no room for complacency, and health improvement work programmes will need to tackle the areas of poor performance, such as:

- failure to provide NHS equivalent primary healthcare and mental healthcare
- delays in transferring mentally ill prisoners to NHS secure services
- failure to detect incipient mental health problems
- not detecting or noticing the weak and mentally frail prisoners and lack of training for prison staff in observing signs of frailty
- professional isolation of clinical staff
- social isolation of inpatients locked up for up to 22 hours a day
- occupational deprivation in inpatient healthcare centres
- no NHS equivalent patients complaints procedure

- increasing numbers of suicides
- poor observation of those at risk
- dirty and depressing environments in some healthcare centres
- staff skill mix inappropriate for patient needs; under-utilisation of nurses' skills.

As stated earlier, there is always a risk that those persons who are hidden away from the community as prisoners will be forgotten. The challenge for nurses is to recognise the risk, to have the courage to intercede on behalf of prisoners' health, and not to tolerate standards that they would not tolerate for their own relatives. Nurses must always remember that each prisoner is a person with his or her own personal story. When a prisoner walks through the gates of a prison, he or she remains all that he or she was on the outside: a father, a mother, a sister, a brother, a child, a farmer, a doctor, a nurse, an accountant, and the loss sustained by imprisonment is profound. The effect of imprisonment on a person's mental health is the proper concern of the nurse who should do everything possible to understand the effects of imprisonment and to limit the damage thereby caused to the individual.

Given the risks inherent in a person being imprisoned, that in the absence of countermeasures deprivation of freedom is intrinsically bad for mental health, and that imprisonment has the potential to cause significant mental harm, the governor and senior management team, together with prison staff and clinicians, have a clear duty to develop preventative measures and healthy regimes for prisoners to promote positive mental health and well-being.

It is easy to feel overwhelmed and lose heart when there is so much to be done. This is why it is important to have someone in post to lead, manage and support staff, as well as putting clinical governance arrangements in place in prisons. But each of us has to start from where we are. The actual truth about the standards of care in a particular prison requires an honest and courageous examination. Having found out the strengths and weakness of the service in relation to the prisoners' assessed needs and having sought prisoners' views, it is important, in the first instance, for the whole clinical team to agree some essential quality standards as part of the clinical governance action plan. Consulting and involving general prison staff is important because most prison healthcare is primary care for prisoners on the residential wings and is not confined to the hospital wings or healthcare centres. Because confinement in prison constitutes a hazard to individual health, especially to mental health, the general prison staff must be made fully aware that preservation of health is the concern of everyone, not only the clinical staff.

Earlier, I described how the government has given top priority to ensuring that in the NHS quality care, as a right for every patient, will be ensured through a system of clinical governance. The NHS is seeking to change its thinking on improving quality by encouraging all the professions towards a coherent aim of making the quality of the patient's experience better in every way. This could be a model for prison governance too, and could usefully be adapted to make the quality of the prisoner's experience the driving force in prisons. At present, there is no quality governance system in the prison service in this way.

The prison service has published a series of performance standards, which are monitored by its own operating standards audit teams. The task of these is to ensure complete compliance with prison operating standards, rules and regulations by regular visits to all establishments. Though there are points of similarity, HMIP's approach to inspection of prisons is different because the Chief Inspector's remit is 'to monitor and report on the treatment of and conditions for prisoners', which essentially means concentrating on the quality of outcomes for prisoners of service delivery within prisons.

During the mid and late 1990s the Chief Inspector and his staff considered how to bring a quality dimension to the inspection of, treatment of, and conditions for prisoners. Following work on the inspectorate's thematic report *Suicide Is Everyone's Concern* (Home Office, 1999), during which wide discussions took place and appropriate literature was reviewed, including the World Health Organization's *Health in Prisons Project* (WHO, 1998), it was decided that the quality imperative was best encapsulated in the concept of healthy prisons. Consequently healthy prison criteria were developed, forming the pillars of quality, guiding the understanding of what a healthy establishment is, and providing a sound basis from which to judge the effect on prisoners of their treatment and conditions. *Health-Promoting Prisons: A Shared Approach* (DOH, 2002) is a further step in exploring the concept of prisons as sources of health awareness.

Providing a healthy environment

It may seem difficult at first to think of or view an institution or organisation as healthy or unhealthy. Perhaps a few definitions from the *Oxford English Dictionary* (OED, 1993) might help. Healthy is defined in the OED as 'possessing good health, sound condition of body; freedom from disease; spiritual and moral soundness; condition of body in respect of its vigour and soundness'. And the OED defines soundness as 'free from any decay or defect, undamaged, unbroken: strong and intellectual on moral qualities, steadfast'. Now if we took each of these and debated the relevance to prisons as organisations, it would probably result in a PhD thesis! We could end up doing a lot of talking and not a lot of doing!

All organisations know why they exist, and what their purpose is. Keeping faith with a clear sense of purpose and translating it into practical realities, with spiritual and moral soundness, for the end-user is a constant challenge. Her Majesty's Prison Service's statement of purpose is clear: 'The Prison Service serves the public by keeping in custody those committed by the courts, our duty is to look after them with humanity and help them to lead law abiding and useful lives on release'. Statements of purpose have to be translated into outcomes and ways of behaving and working to make sure that the spirit of the statement of purpose is evident in the everyday lives of those who work in an organisation.

Her Majesty's Inspectorate of Prisons, in developing a systematic approach to the inspection of prison establishments (Home Office, 2000), has the quality of the prisoner's experience of his or her imprisonment as the core value of the inspection process and it is that which informs the healthy prison criteria. The healthy prison approach to inspection can be best described as the life force, which reaches every aspect of the prisoner's experience. It validates inspection, makes it more accountable and gives the Chief Inspector a quality means of reporting to the public and parliament on the state of our prisons. The healthy prison criteria for inspection combined with the results of prisoners' question-naires about their treatment and conditions provide a solid basis for open and fair inspection judgements.

The healthy prison concept as used in the thematic report *Suicide Is Every-one's Concern* (Home Office, 1999) derived from the World Health Organiza-tion's *Health in Prisons Project* (WHO, 1998), has been further developed by HMIP. The report discusses the concept of healthy prisons, and four criteria, which are used as tests of a healthy establishment, are set out below:

(1)   Prisoners are held in safety.
(2)   Prisoners are treated with respect as fellow human beings.
(3)   Prisoners are expected to improve themselves and are given the opportu-nity to engage in purposeful activity.
(4)   Prisoners are helped to resettle in society and reduce the likelihood of their re-offending.

Because HMIP's focus is on the prisoner's experience of his or her treatment and conditions and the outcomes of that experience, the systematic approach to inspection is framed as a number of outcomes for prisoners under 23 subject areas concerning their treatment, including prison healthcare. Outcomes are defined as the visible or practical positive effect on prisoners as a result of their treatment and conditions.

Expectations is the overall title given to HMIP's *Systematic Approach to Inspecting Prison Establishments* (Home Office, 2000). This publication, setting out a means of inspecting the quality of the outcomes of the prisoner's experience together with the work of the prison service operating standard audit could, over time, form a unified and coherent approach to prison governance as a quality assurance framework for prisons to give life to the prison service's statement of purpose. This would assure those who have the desperate misfortune of losing their liberty, and who are walled off from society, that humanity, dignity, safety and respect prevail in our prisons. It takes time to adjust to the concept of a prison establishment as a healthy or unhealthy place to be in, and it may be confusing particularly for healthcare staff using the same word 'healthy' in two different ways. It may be useful to ask, 'How do the healthy prison criteria apply to prison healthcare?' The answer is: in exactly the same way as they apply to any other aspect of a prisoner's experience of imprisonment. Another question is, 'How healthy is the healthcare service for prisoners?' Prison healthcare has to meet the four healthy prison tests of safety, respect, purposeful activity and resettlement.

Healthy prison outcomes for healthcare should not be confused with clinical outcomes and evidence-based clinical practice, which fall within clinical governance arrangements. *A First Class Service – Quality in the New NHS* (DOH, 1998) sets out four main components of clinical governance as:

(1) clear lines of responsibility and accountability for the overall quality of clinical care
(2) a comprehensive programme of quality improvement activities
(3) clear policies aimed at managing risk
(4) procedures for all professional groups to identify and remedy poor performance.

Clinical governance is the main energiser for maintaining quality at the heart of the NHS including prison healthcare. HMIP's healthy prison 'expectations' include outcomes and expectations for primary care, specialist healthcare, NHS referral, pharmacy, dental healthcare, mental healthcare, inpatient healthcare and maternity services. When developing and reviewing the clinical governance framework in each prison, the inspectorate's outcomes and expectations for healthcare should be taken account of within the framework to form an integrated comprehensive system of quality assurance and make quality healthcare the right of every prisoner.

Summary

The opening of this chapter outlined the low standards prevalent in prison healthcare during the 1990s and the subsequent positive response by ministers to the publication of *Patient or Prisoner?* (HMIP, 1996). Prison healthcare, now, has the leadership of the Prison Health Policy Unit and Task Force, as well as the formal partnership between prison governors and health authorities and a health improvement strategy in every prison. The government's modernisation agenda for the NHS, with quality as a right for every patient, and with an accountable quality assurance system through clinical governance built into health service management, means that there never was a better time for prison healthcare staff to make quality improvement the rightful experience of every prisoner in their care.

References

DOH (1983) *NHS Management Inquiry* (The Griffiths Report). Department of Health, London.
DOH (1997) *The New NHS: Modern – Dependable.* Cm 3807. The Stationery Office, London.
DOH (1998) *A First Class Service – Quality in the New NHS.* Department of Health, London.
DOH (1999) *The Future Organisation of Prison Health Care.* Report by the Joint Prison Service and National Health Service Executive Working Group. Department of Health, London.
DOH (2002) *Health-Promoting Prisons: A Shared Approach. A Strategy for Promoting Health in Prisons in England and Wales.* Department of Health, London.
HMIP (1996) *Patient or Prisoner? A New Strategy for Health Care in Prisons.* Discussion paper. HM Inspectorate of Prisons, London.
HMIP (1998) *Annual Report of HM Inspector of Prisons for England and Wales 1997–98.* Home Office, London.
Home Office (1999) *Suicide Is Everyone's Concern.* Thematic Review by HM Inspectorate of Prisons for England and Wales. Home Office, London.
Home Office (2000) *Expectations – A Systematic Approach to Inspecting Prison Establishments in England and Wales, 2000.* HM Inspectorate of Prisons, Home Office, London.
OED (1993) *The New Shorter Oxford English Dictionary.* Clarendon Press, Oxford.
UKCC (1992) *Code of Professional Conduct for the Nurse, Midwife and Health Visitor,* 3rd edn. United Kingdom Central Council for Nursing, Midwifery and Health Visiting, London.
WHO (1998) *Health in Prisons Project.* Consensus statement on Mental Health Promotion in Prisons. World Health Organization, The Hague.

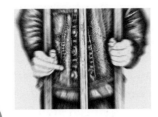

9 Opportunistic Healthcare
A Governor's Perspective

RANNOCH DALY

This chapter provides an important view of prison healthcare from a governor's perspective. It is presented in a different style from that of other chapters because of the message that it is conveying. The prison governor's attitude towards health issues is critical to the delivery of healthcare in any prison. In 13 sections with a concluding vignette, the author describes his views in a unique way. Five appendices contain additional detailed information.

The story begins in May 1999. I was sitting in a pub in Leeds with Hugo Mascie-Taylor. What was I doing there? At least, that's what Mrs Daly asked when I got home.

Armley Gaol

In the city of Leeds no one refers to Leeds Prison as Leeds Prison. Since it opened in 1847 Leeds people have known it as Armley Gaol. In January 1997 I had arrived as the new governor in succession to Tony Fitzpatrick. Armley had been visited in 1996 by the then Minister for Prisons, Ann Widdecombe, to announce the end of slopping out in the prison service. Leeds had been the last prison to slop out. In September 1996 the prison had come to the end of a three-year industrial relations dispute with the Prison Officers' Association (POA), but not by agreement. The management proposals had been imposed.

Healthcare

The Senior Medical Officer (SMO) had moved recently to HMP Wakefield. Among the applicants to be his successor were two of the prison's full-time medical officers: one with nine years' experience of prison medicine and one with three months. The one with three months' experience had been appointed. The one with nine years' experience was now alleging unfair practice in the promotion and appointment of his colleague to be his new SMO boss. The employment tribunal was yet to take place. There were two other doctors, one of whom was subsequently dismissed.

The healthcare staff were a mixture of healthcare officers and nurses in grade E. I learned later that several of these had in fact been recruited as grade D and, regardless of qualifications, had been upgraded following a local industrial relations dispute. There were three Health Care Senior Officers (HCSO), two grade F nurses and one Health Care Principal Officer (HCPO). Another HCPO had reverted to discipline duties in recent management changes and was running one of the residential wings. The SMO, Dr Brendan Carroll, was in charge of the doctors, but all the other healthcare staff had recently been placed in the charge of Chris Walker, a prison service generalist governor with no medical or nursing expertise but with considerable experience in prison management.

The healthcare centre was quite new (completed 1993) but one section was not in use (H2 landing). This was partly because the sanitation system installed was 'electronic unlocking for access to night sanitation' (not the best option for the mentally disordered prisoners who were likely to occupy it) and partly because there appeared to be no funds to staff it. The prison reception was an old, overcrowded rabbit warren of a building that was not fit for purpose but in which the staff were quite proud of their ability to cope. The reception medical examination facilities were primitive and cramped and the examinations were carried out by a part-time locum GP who knew little about the prison, finished working at 7.30 PM, whether she had examined all the prisoners or not, and did no follow-up work with the prisoners after the first night. This was not entirely her fault. She was doing what it said in her contract.

Overcrowding

There was plenty going wrong in healthcare and plenty of scope for anyone working in healthcare to blame someone else. However, this was not my top priority. The main task of 1997 was that, in December, C and D wings were about to reopen after refurbishment (a skimped job as the funding had been halved just before they started). These wings would bring to the prison several hundred additional prisoners but, 'aye there's the rub', nothing for them to do. No work, no education, no training, no programmes, no activity space at all. Just a cell with a toilet in the corner and the prospect of sharing it all day with another prisoner whose criminal record, sexual preferences, violent tendencies and drug habits might be entirely incompatible. Opportunities to urinate and defecate within sight, sound and smell of a complete stranger, and to live and eat in the same space.

CPT

The European Committee for the Prevention of Torture and other Inhuman and Degrading Treatment of Prisoners (CPT) had visited Armley in August 1990 and May 1994. In paragraphs 57 and 58 of the report of their first visit they said:

57.   Overcrowding, lack of integral sanitation and inadequate regime activities would each alone be a matter of serious concern; combined they form a potent mixture. The three elements interact, the deleterious effects of each of them being multiplied by those of the two others. It is a generally recognised principle that people are sent to prison as a punishment, not for punishment. However, many prisoners met by the CPT's delegation understandably perceived their conditions of detention as being in themselves a form of punishment.

In the CPT's view, the cumulative effect of overcrowding, lack of integral sanitation and inadequate regime amounts to inhuman and degrading treatment. This is a matter that needs to be addressed with the utmost urgency.

How should the problem be tackled?

58.   As has been said before by others, the issues of overcrowding and inadequate regimes are inextricably linked.

How to improve regimes in the prisons visited was a constant theme of the delegation's discussions with prison management and prison officers. In the light of everything it heard, the CPT believes that the emphasis must be placed on eliminating overcrowding; remove that and the problem of inadequate regimes – though it will not resolve itself – will at least become solvable.

(CPT, 1991)

On their second visit in May 1994 the CPT noted some improvements, but in paragraph 56 of their report concluded that '... the progress made since the CPT's first visit could be characterised as rather disappointing' (CPT, 1996).

HMCIP 1994

The most recent visit by Her Majesty's Chief Inspector of Prisons (HMCIP) had been on 20–24 June 1994. In the conclusion of his report Judge Stephen Tumin had said:

> 7.01   Conditions for inmates and staff at Leeds were deeply unsatisfactory ... little had changed in conditions for prisoners since the last inspection in 1989.

> 7.11   Leeds staff were trapped in a warehouse with apparently no chance to put things right because of unremitting overcrowding and insufficient activity. ... Leeds has to develop a pride in the service it gives to the public by holding prisoners in decent conditions. There has been little progress towards this objective since the last inspection
>
> (HMCIP, 1994)

All of this, and much more, was explained to me by Tony Fitzpatrick during our handover. The deputy governor and other senior colleagues gave me additional detail. At a Butler Trust awards ceremony at Buckingham Palace in March 2000 Ann Widdecombe told me that in her time as prisons minister she had visited every prison in the country and that Leeds had been the worst.

Changes in healthcare

By the time of the next inspection in September 2000, the Chief Inspector had changed from Judge Tumin to General Ramsbotham. A few things had changed in Armley too. What had changed in healthcare?

- We had increased the total number of main grade healthcare staff to 60.
- We had established and filled posts for:
  - a grade H nurse manager
  - two grade G nurse managers
  - eight grade B nursing assistants
  - nine prison officers within the healthcare team
  - a practice manager at executive officer grade
  - a personal secretary for the senior medical officer
  - a few further posts for a small, dedicated healthcare office support team.
- We had sorted the sanitation on H2 landing and opened it as a drug treatment unit.

- We had extended the remit of the healthcare staff into the main residential wings with a dedicated team of nurses working from wing-based treatment rooms.
- We had dismissed and replaced a full-time medical officer and terminated the contract of the part-time locum GP who worked in reception.
- We had enhanced the reception process by moving some of it into a new first-night centre established in D wing.
- We had ensured that all new receptions were examined in their first four hours in the prison both by a nurse and by a full-time MO in the first-night centre (for an extended account, see Vignette 9.13).
- We had started improving the layout and use of the old reception building.

HMCIP 2000

Much remained to be done both with healthcare and in the wider prison, on overcrowding and on other matters, but Sir David Ramsbotham's opening paragraph said:

> This is a thoroughly good report on the most overcrowded local prison in the country – its actual population of 1,238 being 62% above its Certified Normal Allocation (*sic*) of 770. Of course there is room for improvement in a number of areas – there always will be. But the main point is that the sound foundation laid by the previous governor [Rannoch Daly] is both re-cognised and being exploited by his successor [Stacey Tasker], supported by the area manager, and built on by both management and staff. What is par-ticularly pleasing is to see the responsible and constructive part being played in all this by the POA chairman, secretary and committee. This confirms the importance of the contribution of positive staff associations to the running of prisons, and is a clear indication of what can be achieved if everyone is united by the same aim.
>
> (HMCIP, 2001)

Vignette 9.1

Tension at the top

In 1996 the Senior Medical Officer (SMO) transfers to another prison. Among the applications for promotion to the post are two Medical Offi-cers (MOs) from Armley: one with nine years' experience of prison medicine and one with three months'. The one with three months' experience gets the job. He is Dr Brendan Carroll, a man whose background includes 13 years as a GP in the Leeds area. The MO with nine years' prison experience feels aggrieved and lodges an allegation of unfair treatment with an employment tribunal (ET).

As I arrive, the ET concerning the appointment of the SMO is looming. Working together is becoming increasingly difficult for the SMO and the MO and this is becoming problematic for the rest of the healthcare team. Before, during and after ET, I spend a lot of time talking with the MO and SMO individually and together about the case and about the implications for future team working.

The ET concludes that the selection process had not been unfair.

The SMO and the MO find a *modus vivendi*.

Mrs Daly: This Hugo Mascie-Taylor. Who is he?

Patient or prisoner?

In 1996 Her Majesty's Chief Inspector of Prisons, Sir David Ramsbotham, had initiated a debate about health in prisons in his short discussion paper on prison healthcare *Patient or Prisoner?* (HMIP, 1996). Who should run healthcare in prisons? Should it be the prison service, as it had been for over 100 years, or should it be the health service? Sir David recommended the NHS. HMIP's recommendations are addressed to the Home Secretary, who had to refer this one to the Health Secretary.

There seemed to be two initial conclusions by the NHS. The first was: 'We're not sure about this.' The second was: 'However, let's see what we can do.' Ministers commissioned a further study by a working party under the joint chairmanship of Dr Graham Winyard, Director of Health Services, NHS Executive, and Dr Mike Longfield, Director of Health Care, HM Prison Service.

The group also included HMCIP's medical inspector, Dr John Reed.

FutOrg

In addition to ministerial offices in Whitehall (Richmond House) and a few other HQ buildings in London, the NHS has a large HQ building at Quarry House in Leeds. I remember members of the working party visiting Armley from Quarry House in 1998: Dr Gillian Fairfield and Sir Charles Nightingale – there's a good name for someone who works in the health service. The opening paragraph of their report, *The Future Organisation of Prison Health Care* (commonly known as *FutOrg*) (DOH, 1999b), seemed to echo our conversations during their visit (see Appendix A). The message for the future was quite clear.

- Most prisoners spend only a short time in custody before returning to the wider community.
- They are a high morbidity, high risk section of the population.
- They and their families are otherwise difficult to reach.
- To use time in prison to best effect, a partnership between the prison service and the NHS has advantages for the health of the community.

QEII

The report was to be launched in the QEII Conference Centre in Westminster in June 1999 by Martin Narey, Director-General of the prison service, and Sheila Adam, Deputy Medical Director of the NHS. The next thing that happened to me was a phone call from Gillian Fairfield asking me to speak at the launch conference.

'On what subject?' said I.

'On clinical governance,' said she.

'What's that?' said I.

We shall return to that question later.

Vignette 9.2

A staffing package?

Over a period of several weeks I have one-to-one interviews in private with each of the healthcare staff, from senior medical officer to junior nurse, to assist me (and them) in formulating a strategy for the future. After some deliberation Dr Carroll, Chris Walker and I agree that we should establish three nursing groups (inpatients, drugs unit, and wing-based community nursing team) and we should introduce one H grade and two G grade nurse managers.

It takes several months to get a package together with appropriate grade and skill mix, shift patterns, etc. After several meetings with healthcare staff it becomes clear that they are split on its merits. We are working up towards a ballot, but also working up towards the arrival of the new H and

G grades. Is it fair to introduce three new nurse managers into a staffing and industrial relations tangle not of their making? What a welcome to the prison service that would be.

I decide not to proceed at this stage.

Mrs Daly: Have you met Hugo before?

Inequalities in health

In May 1999 I was in Blackwells, the academic bookshop in Leeds, buying some flat Ordnance Survey maps for a mural on the wall next to the stairs at home. My attention drifted into unfamiliar territory – the medical textbooks. I remembered that I had been asked to address a major prison health conference on the subject of clinical governance. Was there a simple publication called *Teach Yourself Clinical Governance*? No, there was not (though there is now – see below).

But, in the way these things happen, my eye was caught by another publication, *Inequalities in Health* by Sir Douglas Black, former Chief Scientist at the Department of Health. Despite an initially frosty reception by ministers (*Lancet*, 6 September 1980), the Black report is a classic of public health analysis that has shaped thinking among public health professionals ever since.

The Health Education Council had commissioned an update in 1987 by Margaret Whitehead, *The Health Divide*. What I had spotted was a Penguin omnibus edition, including both Black and Whitehead (Black, 1980; Whitehead, 1992). Was this just a historical curiosity? Was there anything here about social exclusion? Was there anything about health deprivation? About equal access to health and healthcare? There was – in spades.

In her Chapter 9, 'Action on inequalities: policy in the caring services' (Whitehead, 1992), Margaret Whitehead notes (cited from Griffiths, 1991) that 'a targeted, community-based approach alone will reach social groups which need the most support – any other strategy could waste scarce resources'. In only 20 pages (pp. 355–74) she reviews a wide range of studies showing that, with a little bit of energy and thought, healthcare can be targeted at those who need it most and who otherwise might be hard to find (for a list of 38 examples, see Appendix B).

In 1997 the government commissioned a further update by Sir Donald Acheson (Acheson, 1998). His report contains 39 recommendations about the links between health and:

- poverty
- education
- housing
- employment
- nutrition
- ethnicity
- gender
- older people
- transport
- mothers, children and families
- young people and adults of working age
- the NHS.

There is no specific mention of prisons or prisoners in Acheson's report, but we know from other sources that most prisoners and their families come from conditions of poor educational attainment, poor housing and poor employment records. For many, their pattern of consumption of food, drink and drugs could hardly be described as nutritious. There is a disproportionately high number of prisoners from the ethnic minorities. Prisoners are mainly in their teens, twenties and thirties so have many young children. We know from examining prisoners that, compared with others of the same age, they are of poor health. Prisoners and their families come from those communities experiencing social exclusion and health deprivation. Consequently, Acheson makes many comments relevant to our work in prisons. For example:

Suicide

There is a steep social class gradient in deaths from suicide. In 1991–93, rates for men were 4 times higher in social class V than in social class I. Our policies aim to reduce the causes of social exclusion which lead to despair and to improve mental health services for people who are already mentally ill. Detailed evidence in support of these recommendations is given at appropriate points in the preceding text.

34.   We *recommend* policies which reduce the excess mortality from accidents and suicide in young men. Specifically:
- We recommend policies which improve the opportunities for work and which ameliorate the health consequences of unemployment (recommendation 8).
- We recommend policies which improve housing provision and access to health care for both officially and unofficially homeless people (recommendation 11).

- We recommend policies to prevent suicide among young people, especially among young men and seriously mentally ill people (recommendation 24).
- We recommend policies which reduce alcohol-related ill health, accidents and violence, including measures which at least maintain the real cost of alcohol (recommendation 26.5).

(Acheson, 1998, p. 107)

Whitehead coins the phrase 'opportunistic health care' and quotes Dowling (1983): '… when attention is given to the lifestyles and needs of the parents, most families can be contacted, often with surprising ease'.

'Opportunistic' healthcare? Prison as an opportunity? Why not?

Vignette 9.3

Disappointment

With the growing numbers of nurses and nurse-qualified healthcare officers, the future will require nurse-qualified healthcare managers. The healthcare principal officer at Armley is not nurse-qualified. He is assured of a continuing role at the prison either in operations or in residence. After nearly 20 years in healthcare this is not his first preference. He is disappointed but he understands and he accepts with good grace.

Mrs Daly: How did you first hear of Hugo Mascie-Taylor?

Prisoners and their families

The number of people in prison during recent years has been about 65 000. In the most recent year for which the figures have been published (1999) the number who came into prison was 135 100 (Home Office, 2000). Thus, by simple arithmetic, the average length of stay in prison must be slightly less than six months.

However, some people come to prison and stay there for much longer than six months, sometimes for many years. Thus, the average covers both a minority that is in prison for longer than six months and a majority that is in prison for less than six months.

Less than six months = 80%

Of the 135 100 people who came to prison in 1999, only about 25 000 (less than 20%) could expect to be there for longer than six months. The other 110 000 people received into prison in 1999 (more than 80% of the total) were there for less than six months. Whatever we do with prison receptions, more than 80% are back in the community within six months. Less than 20% of the effect accrues to the prison: more than 80% accrues to the community (for a graph showing lengths of time spent in prison, see Appendix C).

Who are prisoners?

Ninety-five per cent of prisoners are male. Most of them are young, in their teens, twenties and early thirties. Most of them have partners (sometimes more than one) and children. Most of these children are of school or pre-school age. Taken together with their partners and children, the 135 000 people coming into prison each year represent at least half a million men, women and children: about 1% of the population.

Are prisoners healthy?

The fact that they are mostly young might lead one to expect that prisoners will be mostly healthy, but they are mostly not. The 1% of the population who either come to prison themselves or whose parent or partner comes to prison live predominantly in the parts of our towns and cities where health and access to healthcare is poorest.

Tooth-brushing, regular exercise, healthy eating patterns, non-smoking, the drinking of water, no abuse of illegal substances, the absence of stress, healthy partners, good quality housing, stable employment – are these what we associate with prisoners? Are these the circumstances in which their partners and children are living?

If the condition of most prisoners on reception is any guide, the answer is no. Whether through psychoses, neuroses, drug abuse or a combination of these and other conditions over 80% of all prison receptions have some form of mental disorder (Singleton, 1998). Prison health needs assessments (HNAs – see below) shed more light on the ill health of prisoners and, by implication, their families.

For the prisoner, we will try to provide a proper health service in the prison, but:

- Who makes the strenuous efforts needed to provide healthcare to prisoners' children?
- Can you use the prison as an opportunity to enhance family health?
- You can put the prisoner in touch with health professionals. How can you do this for the prisoner's family?

When we can answer those questions we will be entitled to believe that the prison is making an active contribution to the partnership.

Vignette 9.4

B grades

An analysis of the healthcare staff workload and the appropriate skill mix at Armley identifies a case for some nursing assistants at grade B – possibly up to ten.

    Grading guidance is consulted and job descriptions are prepared but discussion with local Prison Officers' Association representatives establishes that there is no national level agreement about nursing assistants. Is this an obstacle or an opportunity?

Mrs Daly: This Hugo-Mascie Taylor. Who introduced you?

Partnership

Following the publication of *The Future Organisation of Prison Health Care* (DOH, 1999b) the partnership of the prison service with the NHS has taken some time to establish. As successors to the Directorate of Health Care in the Prison Service two teams were established – the Prison Health Policy Unit (PHPU) and the Prison Health Task Force (PHTF). The partnership feature of these units is best expressed by two phenomena unusual in Whitehall. They

- appear in the management structure charts of both the prison service and of the NHS, and
- are reponsible to both the Minister for Prisons and Probation in the Home Office (Paul Boateng, succeeded by Beverley Hughes) and to the Minister of State at the Department of Health (Lord Hunt, succeeded by Jacqui Smith).

PHPU/TF

The PHPU works like a traditional policy team in a Whitehall department drafting documents for the minister, for parliament, for the service and the public. The non-traditional feature is working for two separate ministers in two separate departments.

The PHTF has a specific brief to establish the foundations and mechanics of the partnership through prisons, their staff, governors and area managers and through primary care groups and trusts, other trusts (such as mental health), health authorities and NHS regional offices. During 2001 a small task force team was established in each of the eight NHS regions to work jointly for prison area managers and NHS regional directors in order to carry the partnership forward.

The heads of the PHPU (Felicity Harvey) and of the PHTF (John Boyington) were both appointed in March 2000.

Felicity Harvey (PHPU)

Felicity is a doctor and microbiologist who has moved into health administration at senior level in Whitehall. She has been Private Secretary to the former Chief Medical Officer (Sir Kenneth Calman). After completing an MBA she became Head of Quality Management for the NHS, laying the foundations for the National Institute for Clinical Excellence (NICE), the Commission for Health Improvement (CHI) and practice of clinical governance throughout the NHS.

John Boyington (PHTF)

John started off as a psychiatric nurse and worked his way up through senior nurse and nurse manager posts to nurse director and to Chief Executive of Leicester Community and Mental Health Trust, the largest of its type in the country, with over 6000 employees.

Projects

A number of specific projects have been established jointly by the PHPU/TF. The report *Nursing in Prisons* (DOH, 2000a) was published in October 2000 and the consequent implementation work is being taken forward by the Prison Service Director of Nursing, Lindsay Bates. A similar project on prison medical staff was presented its report in December 2001. The Prison Service Medical Director, Cliff Howells, will take the lead on implementation of those recommendations accepted by ministers.

Prison Health Projects: 2000

- Health services: pharmacy, dentistry, primary care.
- Mental health, reception screening, health promotion, harm minimisation, substance misuse.
- Health staffing: nursing, medical staff.
- Health management: health information systems (IT), performance monitoring, clinical governance.

Further work for the PHPU/TF over the three years 2001–2004 includes:

- £35m for improvements in prison healthcare buildings and facilities
- £17m to health authorities (£2m, £5m and £10m in 2001–2002, 2002–2003 and 2003–2004 respectively) to build up to a total of 300 staff to deliver CPA (the care programme approach) in mental health in-reach work in prisons (see below – mental health)

There seems to be no shortage of new work requiring new projects. Details of the PHPU and PHTF and prison health developments were sent to all prisons and health authorities in the *Prison Health Handbook* in September 2000 (DOH, 2000b), and information is updated every three months in the *Prison Health Newsletter*.

Vignette 9.5

An employment tribunal

To enable the full-time medical officers to carry out the reception health screening we have to terminate the contract of the part-time locum GP who has done it up to now. At an employment tribunal (ET) she alleges discrimination on the grounds of sex and race – she is Asian. We argue that there is an operational and a clinical need to have reception health screening done on reception by full-time medical officers who know the prison and its personnel, and who can follow up their findings within a few days. We also argue that our procedures were quite proper, in accordance with her contract and with employment law (for example, with regard to the period of notice given).

Mrs Daly: Was anyone else there, or was it just you and this Hugo?

Health needs assessment

In their partnership with the prisons the NHS people needed somewhere to start.

- Who are these 135 000 people coming into prison each year?
- What are their health needs?
- What do we already know?
- How do we find out more?

Expertise in health needs assessments lies with Professor Andrew Stevens and his colleagues in the Department of Public Health and Epidemiology at the University of Birmingham. The academic library shelves groan under the weight of huge tomes of *Health Needs Assessments* (Stevens *et al.*, 2000).

Toolkit

The PHPU/TF commissioned the Birmingham team to prepare a health needs assessment of the prison population as a whole and to provide a toolkit with which individual prisons could assess their own population in conjunction with their local health authority (Stevens *et al.*, 2000). Of course, prison healthcare professionals already knew a great deal in this area but it had not been gathered together and analysed in such a systematic manner. The first health needs assessments (HNAs) in individual prisons were completed in March 2001 and formed the basis of annual prison health improvement programmes (HImPs) during 2001–2002.

Professor Stevens' HNA of the prison service runs to 150 pages and draws upon over 200 previously published sources. There are many nuggets of useful information. I will ask the reader to consider only two – beds and primary care contacts.

Beds

In England and Wales the number of healthcare beds per 1000 of the population is 5. In the prisons of England and Wales the number of healthcare beds per 1000 prisoners is 29. Compared to the community, per head, the prisons have almost six times as many healthcare beds.

Primary care contacts

Counting doctors, nurses and healthcare officers as primary care staff and counting how frequently prisoners have contact with them and comparing that with equivalent figures from the community, what do we find? In prisons, of course, all prisoners have an initial contact in reception. They also see nursing staff to receive medication which, in the community, they might obtain from the chemist's shop in the high street and administer to themselves (self-care) or through a family member (informal care). However, the comparison produces stunning results. For every occasion in the community on which men or women of comparable age have contact with a doctor, prisoners have contact five times. For every occasion in the community in which men of comparable age have contact with a nurse (about once every three years), male prisoners have contact 77 times (about once a fortnight). For women the comparable figure is 197 times – more than once a week (Stevens *et al.*, 2000, pp. 69–70). Thus, if women in the community see a healthcare professional once every six months, women in prison see a healthcare professional once every 23 hours. And these figures are just the averages.

An HImP question

For discussion at your next prison health improvement plan (HImP) steering group meeting: 'In the community we encourage healthy lifestyles, self-care and informal care. In the prisons how can we avoid doing the opposite?'

Many of the informational nuggets from Professor Steven's HNA of the prisons can be used quite easily as the basis for useful exercises. (For a team exercise based on 'beds' and 'primary care', see Appendix D.)

Vignette 9.6

A budget blow

We have managed to carve out of our existing budget enough money to plan for next year how to open and staff H2 landing as a drug treatment unit. We then learn that, owing to government financial policy, our budget is to be cut next year by a similar amount. The plan is put on the shelf.

However, a bid for funds for a drugs unit under the comprehensive spending review (CSR) is successful. The plan comes back off the shelf and is implemented. This includes replacing the electronic unlocking (for access to night sanitation) with in-cell toilets.

Mrs Daly: This meeting with Hugo Mascie-Taylor. Did it have a specific purpose?

What clinical governance is not

There are two problems with clinical governance. The first is the word 'clinical' and the second is the word 'governance'.

Clinical

Like many medical words 'clinical' derives from the language of the ancient Greeks. A *kline* was a bed. A *klinikos* was a person who took to his bed, and it could also refer to the person who looked after the people in bed. An interesting adaptation of the term in mediaeval times was the phrase 'clinical conversion', which referred to a person being baptised into the church on their deathbed. 'Clinical skills' are, originally, those of tending to the ill who are confined to bed (*klinike* – the clinical art).

The meaning of 'clinic' as a place where specific medical skills or expertise might be found or practised, is a comparatively modern meaning of the term that developed during the late nineteenth century. An even more modern meaning of the term is its use as a taboo, bogeyman phrase by the medical profession to ward off the layman. George Bernard Shaw said, 'all professions are conspiracies against the laity'. In this respect the word 'clinical' has been one of the more powerful terms with which doctors (and nurses too) protect their territory. In this field our language abounds with phrases such as 'that's a matter of clinical judgement' and 'that's confidential, it's a clinical matter' and 'you can't tell me what to do on clinical matters; I'll take it up with the NMC', and so on.

'Clinical' speaks of technical skill and expertise acquired through long study, practice and apprenticeship. Which is fine. I have no wish to tell doctors which drugs to prescribe for which illnesses or how to carry out hip replacements. However, given a few facts, any layman is perfectly capable of asking a doctor why their prescription seems to be radically different from that of most of their colleagues. Or asking why one surgeon's hip replacement patients seem to be able to walk quite well and the patients of another surgeon don't. Or distinguishing between a clean ward and a dirty ward. Good doctors and nurses are delighted if someone shows an interest.

Governance

The word 'governance' is equally off-putting. It has a somewhat old-fashioned ring to it. It looks like the word 'government' but it's different so, presumably it means something similar to government but not quite the same. In prisons the person in charge is called the governor and we say that they 'govern', but we never say that they practise 'governance'; so it must mean something different from that term too. It was used in the title of a book by Harold Wilson called *The Governance of Britain* (Wilson, 1976). I remember that reviewers at the time found it a rather artificially high-flown term. It does sound a bit eighteenth centuryish, don't you think? Perhaps the sort of affectation in which you would not wish to indulge.

Vignette 9.7

A ballot

The new H and G grades have been in post for some months and have reworked the old package of staffing arrangements in consultation with me, the doctors, the healthcare staff, the POA, colleagues in other parts of the prison, Old Uncle Tom Cobleigh and all.

   Because of the implications for reception and for wing-based nursing the POA reach the conclusion that a ballot of the whole prison is appropriate. It is a matter for them but, as it happens, I agree.

   The package is voted in.

Mrs Daly: When you were talking with Hugo Mascie-Taylor what were you talking about?

What clinical governance is

Corporate governance

'Corporate governance' was a vogue phrase in the business circles of the City of London in the early 1990s. Concern had grown on the stock exchange about the accountability of company directors to their shareholders, about the extent to which shareholders had sufficient detailed knowledge of the company's financial affairs and, in particular, about the duties and responsibilities of directors.

   The recommendations of Cadbury (1992), Greenbury (1995) and Hampel (1998) were consolidated into what became known as the 'combined code';

setting out various expectations of the directors of listed companies. At this point some ingenious individual came up with a cunning plan. The code was not made compulsory. However, to be listed on the stock exchange, a company either had to state in its annual report that it operated in compliance with the code or include a statement of those elements of the code that did not apply and why the company had decided not to apply them. Needless to say, there was no great rush to declare oneself non-compliant. As Eric Morecambe used to say: 'Get out of that. You can't, can you?'

Management

Corporate governance was a move in the direction of accountability and transparency. Another movement had been growing in the NHS for some years. Many would say that it was inevitable from the foundation of the NHS in 1948 but, if that was the case, it did not become manifest till much later. This movement was the rise of the manager and the rise of management.

The welfare state

In 1948 there were doctors and there were nurses and there were a few civil servants dealing with health and there seemed to be an assumption that, the welfare state having been established, they were best left to get on with it. The medical profession had not been keen on the NHS and had had to be 'brought along'. Nurses were vocationally dedicated and while they might have to be terrorised by matron (Hattie Jacques) they did not have to be 'managed'. Civil servants were there to get the money out of the Treasury. Patients would be compliant and grateful. Where did responsibility lie for making decisions? Who made them? Who didn't? Where was the money actually going? Was it improving health? Many of these were questions it would have occurred to few people to ask.

Commerce

In 1948 management was not the profession it is today. There had been agricultural and industrial revolutions in the eighteenth and nineteenth centuries in Europe, in the USA and in a few other countries. In the early twentieth century a few individuals had written on what we would now call management (such as Frederick W. Taylor, Chester Barnard, Alfred P. Sloan, Lyndall Urwick, Elton Mayo) but the marketing and productivity revolutions of the post-war era were still ahead. Management as a subject for study, teaching and application (and for shelves in bookshops) was a concept confined to a few academics and

entrepreneurs: particularly a few Americans working to rebuild Japanese industries after Hiroshima and Nagasaki had ended the war in the east (W. Edwards
Deming, Joseph Juran, etc.).

Confronted by the Japanese success with cars and consumer goods, the West
emulated the American example. The more systematic approach to quality in
management was adopted by other manufacturing industries and by service
industries (such as hotels, airlines, holiday companies, etc.). The business community was driven by profit and by business survival. Management worked
(Kennedy, 1993).

Government

Government is less dependent on the disciplines of the market and has other
non-market pressures with which to cope. Value-for-money management
caught on more slowly in the public sector but gradually the point became
accepted in the public sector too – if you could manage public services more
effectively you could make the same money do more, or even 'do more with
less'. The evidence of the past few years is that all political parties in Britain now
profess their commitment to management and value-for-money in their
approach to government. A principal strand of argument between British political parties now is the question of who is the better manager: of the economy, of
transport, of education, of law and order, etc.

Health management

The NHS has been feeling the effects of these wider developments. Whether
through the internal health market, the development of health centres, GP
fundholders, trusts or performance targets the pressures to manage healthcare
have been growing. Many doctors and nurses have preferred to work exclu-
sively in direct contact with patients (clinical skills) but many others have developed management skills and, on either a part-time or a full-time basis, become
effective managers of their services. For senior people in the health service an
MBA is becoming *de rigeur*.

Patients

Patients are not as compliant now as was expected in 1948. The population as a
whole is better educated (about 40% of 18-year-olds go to a university), better
informed (the media has expanded tremendously), more demanding and more
able to express those demands, if necessary through litigation (the rise of the

'compensation culture'). The spectacular misdemeanours of some doctors, whether deliberate or unintended (Harold Shipman, the Bristol babies' heart surgeons, etc.) has raised the profile of the medical profession further. Neither patients nor government are willing to leave the medical profession accountable only to themselves. Wise heads within medicine have judged that their best way forward is openness and to take their patients with them.

Clinical governance

The trends towards transparency, accountability, management and openness all find expression in clinical governance. In layman's terms this means improving healthcare openly. It means taking the principles and practices of quality assurance, quality improvement and customer focus that have been developed in the manufacturing and service industries, and applying them to health services. It means:

- looking for evidence and acting upon it
- comparing your practice with others
- counting things
- monitoring and indicators
- audits and surveys
- having priorities and action plans
- personal objectives and team objectives
- staff development and training
- continuing professional development
- tackling poor performers
- improving the suitability of your buildings and equipment
- taking responsibility
- being open with individual patients and with patients as a group.

It is no different from managing all the other areas of the prison for which the governor is responsible but in which he/she has no particular expertise. It is like managing the catering or the visits or anything else. It has its own particular healthcare wrinkles but the principles are the same.

The more I think about it the more it seems possible that prisons could become centres of excellence in the practice of clinical governance. We've been doing governance in other areas for years. Now we need to do governance in healthcare.

Dr Jamie Harrison (a medical officer at HMP Frankland) and Professor Tim van Zwanenberg (University of Newcastle) have edited an excellent short book called *Clinical Governance in Primary Care*, which is eminently applicable to prisons (van Zwanenberg & Harrison, 2000).

Vignette 9.8

Dismissing a doctor

One of our doctors had been recruited by HQ as a medical officer and allocated to HMP Leeds in 1995. In 1996 Armley staff learned from a newspaper article that he was in trouble with the GMC over his previous practice in Derby and required supervision, training and review by the GMC at intervals of 12 months, sometimes 6 months. It would have been perfectly proper to terminate his contract in 1996 but instead it was decided to try to provide the supervision and training. After two years he was making no progress. In considering the next step we sent to HQ for his personnel file and discovered that he had not been wholly frank about the GMC position on his recruitment. I suspended him.

There was a factual inquiry, a disciplinary hearing, a dismissal, an appeal within the prison service, a further appeal to the Civil Service Appeals Board and an employment tribunal case, settled out of court for less than the cost of defending.

Mrs Daly: Was this discussion with Hugo Mascie-Taylor just out of personal interest or something to do with the prison?

Performance assessment framework

If clinical governance is about improving things, which things are we aiming to improve? How does the NHS describe its performance aspirations? Are they of any relevance to prison health?

The Performance Framework for the NHS set out in *A First Class Service: Quality in the New NHS* (DOH, 1998) focuses on six main areas:

(1) health improvement
(2) fair access to services
(3) effective delivery of appropriate healthcare
(4) efficiency
(5) patient and carer experience
(6) health outcomes of NHS care.

(DOH, 1998, p. 64. For details of these six areas, see Appendix E)

As illustrations of some of the implications, consider:

- *Fair access*; for example geographical. An implication:
  - — Why is provision better in one local prison than in another?
- *Appropriate healthcare*; for example delivered by appropriately trained and educated staff. An implication:
  - — Are yours?
  - — Have you checked?
  - — What further training would be beneficial?
- *Patient experience*; for example patient involvement, good information and choice. An implication:
  - — Choice is difficult to provide in a prison, which means extra emphasis on information and involvement.
- *Outcomes*; for example reducing levels of risk factors. An implication:
  - — Carry out risk assessments of individuals and of their living and working environment.

Vignette 9.9

Finding a doctor

The area Principal Medical Officer (PMO) was visiting and mentioned that a senior medical officer in another prison was struggling because his governor wanted him to spend more time managing healthcare and he wanted to spend more time seeing patients. I had worked with this doctor before so I knew his managerial interest to be low but his clinical skills to be high. We were carrying a vacancy for a doctor (see Vignette 9.8).
We solved three problems at once:

- At Armley we filled our vacancy.
- At the other establishment the governor was free to pursue his alternative plans for the development of healthcare in his establishment.
- The doctor could spend all his time attending to patients at Armley.

Mrs Daly: This conversation with Hugo Mascie-Taylor. What was the connection with prisons?

National service frameworks

Standards for the delivery of healthcare in the NHS are set out in a series of national service frameworks (NSFs). The first two were on coronary heart disease and mental health. These are substantial documents. The NSF on mental health runs to 150 pages plus an executive summary of 30 pages (DOH, 1999a).

The programme of NSFs is part of the government's agenda to drive up quality and reduce unacceptable variations in health and social services. In the NHS, standards will be:

- set by the National Institute for Clinical Excellence and the NSFs
- delivered by clinical governance, underpinned by professional self-regulation and lifelong learning
- monitored by the Commission for Health Improvement, the new National Performance Assessment Framework and the National Survey of Patients.

NSF – mental health

In the mental health NSF there are seven standards in five areas.

- *Standard 1*   Mental health promotion
- *Standards 2 and 3*   Primary care and access to services
- *Standards 4 and 5*   Effective services for people with severe mental illness
- *Standard 6*   Individuals who care for people with mental health problems
- *Standard 7*   Action necessary to achieve the target to reduce suicides

In each of these areas the NSF sets out a rationale, a service model, performance assessment criteria and the lead roles and responsibilities (health authority, primary care group, etc.).

Primary care

For example, in the area of 'Primary care and access to services', performance will be assessed at national level by:

- A long term improvement in the psychological health of the population as measured by the National Psychiatric Morbidity Survey.
- A reduction in suicide rates.
- The extent to which the prescribing of antidepressants, antipsychotics and benzodiazepines conforms to clinical guidelines.
- Access to psychological therapies.

- Experience of service users and carers, including those from the black and minority ethnic communities.

(DOH, 1999a, p. 10)

Preventing suicide

As another example, the NSF models in preventing suicide direct the NHS agencies specifically to work with staff in prisons: 'Local health and social care communities will help to prevent suicides by delivering the service models set out in this National Service Framework.' The NHS agencies should also (DOH, 1999a, p. 160; my emphasis):

- support prison staff in preventing suicides among *prisoners* including those on remand
- ensure that *staff* are competent to assess the risk of suicide especially among individuals most vulnerable, including people who have self-harmed or attempted suicide, individuals with serious drug and alcohol problems, or those in contact with specialist mental health services, and know what action to take if they are concerned
- develop local systems for suicide *audit* to learn lessons and take any necessary action.

Vignette 9.10

Director-General

In March 2000 the Director-General, Martin Narey, visits HMP Leeds. 'Show me your worst,' he says.

We do. Within weeks money becomes available from the area manager to refurbish visits and reception prior to the visit of HMCIP later that year.

Mrs Daly: Your meeting with Hugo Mascie-Taylor. Was it any use?

Performance indicators

In July 2000 the NHS published their second annual set of performance indicators (DOH, 2000c).

Hospital trusts

Outcomes are given for the performance of 181 hospital trusts in 1998/99 on seven clinical indicators (CIs).

- Deaths in hospital within 30 days of surgery (all ages)
  — CI 1A: emergency admissions
  — CI 1B: non-emergency admissions
- Deaths in hospital within 30 days of admission with
  — CI 2: hip fracture (ages 65+)
  — CI 3: heart attack (ages 34–75)
  — CI 4: emergency readmission to hospital within 28 days of discharge from hospital (all ages)
- Discharge from emergency admission to usual place of residence
  — CI 5: within 56 days following a stroke (ages 50+)
  — CI 6: within 28 days following a hip fracture (ages 65+)

On each indicator the average for England is shown and all the trusts are shown in rank order from the highest to the lowest. Just as the prison service groups prisons by type to give reasonable comparability between establishments of very different character (for example local prisons, Category Bs, Cs or Ds, young offender institutions, etc.), in the NHS trusts are grouped into clusters of similar type:

- 26 small/medium acute trusts
- 42 large acute trusts
- 36 very large acute trusts
- 23 acute teaching trusts
- 55 multi-service trusts.

Heart attacks

Consider, as an example, clinical indicator 3 (heart attacks). Within 30 days of emergency admission with a heart attack to the 42 large acute hospitals the average death rate is 9%. The lowest death rate is Good Hope Hospital with 3.5%. The highest death rate is North Middlesex with 16%. Why the difference?

Health authorities

Outcomes are also given for 99 health authorities against 49 indicators under the six areas of the performance assessment framework mentioned on page 156 (and see Appendix E).

Health improvement

Consider, for example, the highest, lowest and average scores for the seven indicators of 'health improvement':

- Deaths from all causes, ages 15–64
  (lowest score West Surrey 70, English average 90, highest score Manchester 150)
- Deaths from all causes, ages 65–74
  (lowest score West Sussex 70, English average 88, highest score Liverpool 121)
- Deaths from cancer
  (lowest score Barnet 115, English average 135, highest score Manchester 190)
- Deaths from circulatory diseases, ages 35–74
  (lowest score West Surrey 95, English average 140, highest score Manchester 200)
- Suicide rates
  (lowest score Barking 5.5, English average 9, highest score Manchester 15)
- Deaths from accidents
  (lowest score Portsmouth 11, English average 16, highest score Manchester 25)
- Serious injury from accidents (>3 days in hospital)
  (lowest score Kingston 220, English average 310, highest score Liverpool 430)

There is an obvious disparity between the industrial northern cities and the leafy, southern counties. What is the cause? What could be done about it?

Benzodiazepines

There is a broad consensus within the NHS that prescribing of benzodiazepines 'should be kept to a minimum' (DOH, 2000c, p. 30). The average prescription rate for England is 16. The lowest is Herefordshire with 9. The highest is Manchester with 32.

   Is there a connection between the high rate of prescribing of benzodiazepines in Manchester and the high rate of suicide? If so, what is the connection? Is one the cause of the other? If so, which is cause and which effect?

Indicators

These are just a few of the questions that can be prompted by gathering some healthcare facts together and pondering their significance. We are doing much the same in the prison service with the development of indicators on security, regimes, staffing and a wide range of other subjects.

Published health indicators enable health service managers to identify priorities openly with data that is available to staff, patients and the public. This creates obvious problems for those at the wrong end of the scale as it highlights their apparent deficiencies. It may also create problems for those whose performance looks to be at the better end of the scale but for whom closer scrutiny may reveal that not all is as rosy as at first glance. (More than one manager has been sacked for misrepresenting the position with inaccurate statistical returns.)

We can devise better indicators and more indicators (or perhaps – 'Better indicators would lead to fewer indicators? Discuss.') but I see no prospect of indicators being de-invented. Both patients and staff will have to find ways of making them more useful.

Prison indicators

Are prison service indicators better? Is the prison service further forward in terms of relevance, comprehensiveness or utility? What indicators would be most informative on the subject of prison health?

Vignette 9.11

Prison officers in the healthcare team

We had filled a few healthcare officer (HCO) vacancies from E grade nurses who chose to regrade. However, these are not enough to fill all the vacancies. We examine whether prison officers without HCO training could fill some of these posts. We think that they could. We advertise within the prison. There are nine vacancies. There are sufficient applicants that we have to sift and interview as part of the selection process.

An interesting consequence is that when these officers join the healthcare team it is noticed that several of the existing HCOs are, by comparison, a bit rusty on their custodial skills and have to do some catching up. It is an indicator of continuing tensions between nurses and HCOs within the healthcare team that a number of the nurses find this highly amusing.

Mrs Daly: What exactly did you get out of this meeting with Hugo Mascie-Taylor?

Primary care

In conversations with health professionals over the past year or so I have found it instructive, when the phrase 'primary care' crops up, to ask them what they mean by the term. What has been instructive is the extent to which many pause before replying, then look puzzled and then find themselves in some difficulty trying to explain a term that they have been using for many years. The replies, when they come, are not all consistent with one another. Why?

1948

In 1948 many GPs worked single-handed using their own home as the surgery and with assistance only from their wife, who might be the receptionist or the nurse or both. There were few group practices and few other people working in general practice. There were also very few women GPs in 1948, but I understand that among medical students qualifying as GPs women are now the majority. During the 1950s the formation of the Royal College of General Practitioners encouraged some collective and organised thinking about general practice and provided a forum within which new ideas and practices could be considered and spread.

Practice nurse

A small number of district nurses became 'attached' to GP practices during the 1950s and 1960s. After the Family Doctors Charter of 1966 provided a subsidy of 70% of the cost of attached staff, the numbers grew more rapidly. The general practice-nursing role expanded into preventive work (such as coronary artery disease prevention, cervical cytology, well-man and well-woman clinics) and into chronic disease management (such as asthma, diabetes and hypertension). The practice nurse was being invented.

Other staff

The range of services available from GP practices also expanded with dieticians, speech therapists, chiropodists, community psychiatric nurses and counsellors. Some of these provided services from the health authority and some were employed directly by the doctors but they all increased the variety of provision from the GP practice.

Health centres

The surgery moved away from the doctor's house into a new type of building: the health centre. General practitioners tended to form small partnerships to share the accommodation available in health centres and to use the growing range of services that regarded the health centre as their base.

Practice manager

Staffing expanded further with receptionists, secretaries and records clerks and there was a need for all this to be managed by someone. By 1990 books on 'Practice management' were appearing and the new profession of practice nurse (1970s and 1980s) was followed by the even newer profession of practice manager (1990s) (Hasler, 1993).

Non-core services?

An interesting response to the growth in the range of services available in primary care was the production by the General Practitioners Committee of the BMA of guidance for GPs that set out:

- the core services 'which most GPs recognise as being included within core general medical services, and which the generality of GPs are equipped to deliver' (one page); and
- 86 examples of 'non-core services' (six pages).

(BMA, 1996)

In another era, many of these non-core services would not have existed at all and many others would have been provided in hospitals as part of secondary care.

Hospital pressures

However, throughout the post-war period, the pressures had been mounting in the hospitals. As we live longer, particularly beyond the ages of 80 and 90, we make increasing demands on inpatient facilities either for long stays or for repeated short stays. The demand for hospital beds has also grown from our habit of inventing new surgical procedures to solve old problems (heart transplants, artificial hips and other joints, etc.) which need hospital beds for operations and for post-operative recovery. Hospital managers have had to keep looking to identify those for whom a stay in hospital can be shorter or unnecessary.

Patients too express preferences for being at home rather than in a hospital. Day-surgery is becoming increasingly common. Some procedures that used to require hospital admission are now done quite successfully by GPs based in their health centres (for example vasectomy). Some GPs run small cottage hospitals with their own inpatients. They may also provide medical services to long-stay homes (for instance for the elderly) and, of course, to prisons.

Primary care groups/trusts

The previous Conservative government recognised the potential of the growing GP practice to become an independent unit with its own finances and accountability and its own devolved power in deciding upon healthcare directions in the locality. The present Labour government has taken that one step further with GP fundholders becoming primary care groups (PCGs) and, in rapid succession, primary care trusts (PCTs). These are larger groupings, each serving a population of about 100 000 people, with teams of perhaps 40 or 50 GPs plus their growing army of non-GP colleagues.

Healthcare units of this size will be able to expand further their range of activities and staff and to refine further their methods of management (better IT, structured patient consultation, more professionalism in the managers, etc.). They will also find it much easier to engage in partnership working with other agencies about the health impact of decisions in the locality (housing, employment, social care, police, sports and recreation bodies, etc.).

These primary care groups and primary care trusts show the government's ongoing commitment to user-focused services within the public sector, while ensuring that central control over expenditure is strengthened through the NHSE in each of the four devolved UK countries (Sines, 2001).

The Health Act 1999 established the opportunity for community healthcare trusts and fundholding practices to apply for primary care group or primary care trust status. The regional NHSE offices monitor these trusts and their responsibilities are to assess and provide healthcare to the local population. This needs to be done with user participation in the planning stages of such services.

As Sines points out (2001):

This role and function requires that each primary care trust gathers intelligence data or information to advise on actual healthcare needs of the local population and demonstrates inter-professional and inter-agency collaboration (e.g. the formation of seamless links with local authority social services and housing departments). In partnership with central government, targets for healthcare delivery will be set by the NHS Health Authority and NHS Executive commissioners of healthcare and these must be reflected in monitoring review meetings with local providers.

It should be pointed out that these changes are restricted to England and other parts of the UK will make their own particular arrangements for their local services.

What is 'primary care'?

I started this section by observing that the question 'What is primary care?' seemed to provoke a variety of responses. Over the past 50 years primary care has been changing constantly, becoming more complex and more varied. There are platitudinous answers that sound true but not very revealing, for example:

'Primary care is healthcare outside hospitals,' or
'Primary care is what GPs do,' or
'Primary care is the patient's first point of contact with health professionals.'

Attempts at more detailed answers immediately become longer, less easy to grasp and less comprehensive in their accuracy. Primary care is a term that covers a range of healthcare activities; the term is already wide and is expanding further. I find that people are wary of committing themselves to any particular definition of primary care, as they fear that that definition might be too limiting.

Prospects for primary care

If existing trends continue over the next decade or so, it suggests that the health centre and the primary care group are likely to grow further in their significance. Some anticipate an NHS that is primary care-led and have put some effort into working out how that might operate in practice (Meads, 1996). Dr Tom Coffey and some of his colleagues have produced a small booklet setting out a vision for primary care in the year 2009 (Coffey *et al.*, 1999).

I would put it this way.

I anticipate that over the next decade those seeking improvements in the health of the public will increasingly find the source of that improvement not in the hospitals but in primary care. Prisons who do not get on board with their local PCG/PCT will fall further and further behind NHS developments.

Vignette 9.12

Office management

The SMO at Armley had recently been a GP in the Leeds area. He was in the habit of working with a practice manager and an office support team. I asked head of management services to look at what this might mean in prison terms (staff grades, numbers, workload, etc.) It took some time to establish but we achieved an executive officer as practice manager, a personal secretary instead of a typist and a small team of administrative officers and administrative assistants. For the most part they did not invent new work. They took over existing work previously done by nurses and healthcare officers, enabling them to substitute clinical work for clerical work.

Mrs Daly: This Hugo Mascie-Taylor. I think I've got him figured out.

Mental health

In the second half of the twentieth century the prison population in England and Wales rose from about 10 000 in 1940 to about 65 000 prisoners in the year 2000. Over the same period the number of people held in mental hospitals fell from over 150 000 to less than 50 000. As a country, our average performance over the past 50 years has been that each year we have closed 2000 mental hospital places and opened 1000 prison places.

Diversion and transfer

For most of the 1990s the number of people transferred from prison to mental hospital each year was about 800. In addition many people who might otherwise have come into prison were identified in advance at police stations and courts and diverted into residential or community psychiatric care and support.

Psychiatric morbidity

Despite this diversion and transfer activity, levels of mental health problems among prisoners remain high. Studies of the incidence of psychiatric morbidity among prisoners show that 90% of prisoners have some form of mental disorder (including addictions and drug abuse). Will we redefine 90% of the prison population as requiring to be detained in a mental hospital? (And will we subject the mental health laws to the very substantial rewrite that would be necessary to do so?) I doubt it. And I wouldn't recommend it.

Mental health in-reach

It follows, therefore, that if we wish to improve the mental health of those released from prison most of the effort to do so will have to be carried out within the prison as part of prison residential care and preparation for release. Hence the government's announcement in *The NHS Plan* (DOH, 2000d) of 300 additional staff to carry out mental health in-reach work providing CPA (the care programme approach) in prisons.

NHS Plan 2000

The NHS Plan identifies three clinical priorities: cancer, coronary heart disease and mental health.

Mental Health
Prison services (Paragraph 14.36)

At any time some 5000 people with serious mental illness will be in prison. It is important to improve the health screening of those received into custody and to identify and provide treatment for prisoners with mental health problems. Within the new partnerships between the NHS and local prisons, some 300 additional staff will be employed.

By 2004, 5000 prisoners at any time should be receiving more comprehensive mental health services in prison. All people with severe mental illness will be in receipt of treatment, and no prisoner with severe mental illness will leave prison without a care plan and a care co-ordinator.

(DOH, 2000d)

Vignette 9.13

A tale of late evenings (health screening on reception)

The Armley 'development plan' was enshrined in a prison service drawing dated January 1988 showing ambitious plans for expansion and redevelopment. One element was a new reception: another was refurbishment of the wings. Wing A was properly refurbished but owing to cuts in the prison service capital programme the schemes for B, C and D wings were scaled down drastically. C and D wings were due to reopen in December 1997 after their minimal refurbish. What to do with them?

First night centre

We decided that D wing would be the reception/induction wing and that the initial health screening should move from the old reception to the new first-night centre on D1 landing. This introduced disruption to very long-standing work routines. It divided work that needed close co-ordination between staff in reception, D wing and the OCU (observation and classification unit).

This co-ordination did not always work smoothly; the reception process would slow down and sometimes extend later into the evening. On occasion it ran on beyond the normal shift finish at 9 PM. One of the final elements of the reception process was the health screening by the doctor, so they were easy targets for the blame:

Q   'What are we waiting for?'
A   'The doctor's still seeing the receptions.'

Dispute

A formal dispute arose with the POA. This went up to area manager level with one feature being the existing instruction that the doctor should see prisoners on reception 'within 24 hours'.

Q   'Why couldn't this wait till the following day?'
A   'Because we don't want to leave the night staff with unknown quantities.'
   The discussion eventually turned on:

POA   'But a prisoner could commit suicide in the night even after the doctor has seen him.'

Doctor: 'If a prisoner tragically commits suicide on the first night would it be better if that happened *after* he'd seen the doctor or *without* seeing the doctor? Which would you rather tell the family and the coroner?'

The area manager said that he had never seen a doctor at an area dispute meeting before.

Pay

There were occasional, exceptional late evenings after that but the subject blew up significantly about a year later when the POA were in dispute with HQ over their pay settlement. The local POA felt constrained by their legal position not to issue any specific industrial action instructions to their members. A consequence was that their non-specific messages were interpreted variously by different staff in different locations but, broadly speaking, messages such as 'Follow instructions to the letter', 'Don't do anything you feel unsafe with' and 'Do things thoroughly: don't take short-cuts' led to an overall slowing down of the prison routine. Prisoners were late out to court, meals were late, activities were late and reception processes were later than ever. Staff were late off duty most nights for a couple of weeks and the climax was reached with us all standing around the centre till 11.30 PM one night looking at each other and wondering what was going to happen next.

The option was open to me, as the governor, to resolve the matter by settling for compliance with the prison service standard and arranging for the doctor to see receptions 'within 24 hours', the following day. Despite the troubles no one in the management team favoured that course of action. Interestingly, by this time, neither did the staff. Management had to issue new and updated instructions on some matters that previously had worked reasonably well without any instructions at all (such as how to unlock prisoners for meals and manage the queue) or with obsolete instructions (for example replacing rub-down searches of prisoners leaving the workshops with pat-down searches). For the first time we had to produce a written account of how prisoners were to move through each stage of the reception process (a good practice guide).

Lesson

A useful overall lesson for the establishment was that although the operating problems in the prison had been caused by a response to a national issue – the pay award – they had been resolved by local initiative and local discussion.

Mrs Daly: You left a loose thread at the end of the section on 'Patient or prisoner?' saying that you would return to the subject of clinical governance. You have included two sections on clinical governance, but you have not said how you came by that knowledge. I deduce that Hugo Mascie-Taylor was your source.

You also said that Dr Gillian Fairfield from the working party asked you to do the speech on clinical governance so I presume that was what prompted the meeting. Brendan Carroll, the SMO at Armley, has been a GP in the Leeds area for many years so he is the most likely person to have introduced you to Hugo Mascie-Taylor. Who is he?

Me: Hugo Mascie-Taylor is the Medical Director for the Leeds Teaching Hospitals Trust. I thought my meeting with him and Brendan to discuss clinical governance was very productive. But there were also my meetings with Liz Scott.

Mrs Daly: Liz Scott? Meetings?

Me: She's the Director of Public Health for Leeds. She chaired the health needs assessment team for the Leeds prisons (Armley, Wealstun and Wetherby).

Mrs Daly: And it took 12 000 words just to tell me that.

Summary

Working in partnership with the NHS will require the prison service and prison staff to acquire some familiarity with how the NHS goes about its business. This will not be a one-way process. I have tried to tell some tales of Armley prison, which colleagues in the prison service will recognise as 'their' issues. I have also tried to introduce some of the history and language of the NHS and some clues about how it is thinking ahead. As with all dialogue between strangers some of this involves discovering that in many respects we are doing the same things but calling them by different names. I hope that I have done a little to assist in the process of mutual understanding.

Appendix A

The future organisation of prison health care (1999)

Most discussions about prison health care consider prisons as distinct entities which have little relevance for or impact on the wider community. This is no longer appropriate. Currently there are 65 000 people in prison in England and Wales, a figure that has been rising over the past few years and that is projected to continue to rise. The number of people who are received into custody any year is very much larger, being 201 000 (*sic*) persons in 1997. Prisoners are a transient population and most spend only a short time in custody before *returning to the wider community* taking with them their health and social problems. They are a section of the population that may be *difficult to reach* in any other situation and for many a spell in prison represents an opportunity for consistent contact with health services. It makes sense therefore that time in prison should be used as an opportunity to ensure that prisoners receive the best health care possible. This has advantages for both the individual, the community and the NHS. Good health care and health promotion in prisons should help enable individuals to function to their maximum potential on release, which may assist in reducing offending. It should also *reduce morbidity in a high risk* section of the general population with medium and long term reduction in demands on the NHS. Better quality care together with improved links to the NHS are also likely to help prevent acute breakdown and consequent tragic incidents such as homicides or suicides by *people with mental illness*.

Source: DOH (1999b) (my emphases).

Appendix B

38 actions on inequalities: policy in the caring services

Projects on all of the following have been tried and found to be successful in targeting healthcare to the most needy:

- a pregnancy walk-in clinic in the town centre
- an antenatal care project in a factory
- keep-your-own obstetric notes
- community paediatric teams
- extra health visitors
- health-promoting schools

- screening at immunisation for iron deficiency, sickle-cell disease and thalassaemia
- providing 'missing care' lists to health visitors
- audits by community health councils
- respite care
- home-help services
- training materials for health visitors and social workers on the health effects of unemployment
- benefits study pack
- welfare rights advice in GP centres
- clinics at drop-in centres for the homeless
- clinics in hostels
- designating healthcare workers for the homeless
- health workers advice to councils on unfit homes
- planning guidance for public health and planners
- vitamin D supplements in Asian foods
- coronary heart disease (CHD) services for all ethnic groups
- accurate information on ethnic minorities
- informal interpreters
- health advocates
- training materials for health professionals
- avoiding inappropriate advice to smokers
- avoiding inappropriate advice on nutrition
- cervical smears
- postnatal depression
- food co-operatives
- crèches
- tranquilliser dependency
- smoke-free environments
- food and nutrition policies
- differentiated targets by social class and gender
- targeting resources to the most deprived districts, areas and groups
- focus on settings
- outreach work to the target groups.

Source: Black, 1992; Whitehead, 1992.

Appendix C

Lengths of time spent in prison by prisoners received in 1999

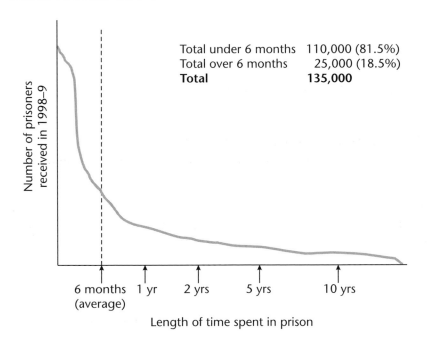

Total under 6 months	110,000 (81.5%)
Total over 6 months	25,000 (18.5%)
Total	**135,000**

Source: Home Office, 2000.

Appendix D

Flipchart exercise
Beds and primary care (times tables)

For a small group (4 to 10 players). Can be health workers but is better with a mixed team including some prison staff with no healthcare background. An interesting exercise for a senior management team.

Question 1   How many healthcare beds per 1000 prisoners are there in your prison?

Question 2   What are the reasons for there to be 6 times as many healthcare beds in prisons as in the community?

Question 3   What are the reasons for contact in male prisons to be 77 times as frequent as in the community? (In female prisons, 197 times?)

When you have used your experience at your prison to list as many reasons as you can, try to allocate the reasons into groups (reasons to do with illness, reasons to do with the prison, reasons which could be changed, etc.).

Incorporate your findings in your prison HImP.

Adapted from Lilley, 1999.

Appendix E
The NHS performance framework

- **Health improvement**
  The overall health of populations, reflecting social and environmental factors and individual behaviour as well as care provided by the NHS and other agencies

- **Fair access**
  The fairness of the provision of services in relation to the need on various dimensions:
  — geographical
  — socio-economic
  — demographic (age, ethnicity, sex)
  — care groups (for example, people with learning difficulties)

- **Effective delivery of appropriate healthcare**
  The extent to which services are:
  — clinically effective (interventions or care packages are evidence-based)
  — appropriate to need
  — timely
  — in line with agreed standards
  — provided according to best practice service organisation
  — delivered by appropriately trained and educated staff

- **Efficiency**
  The extent to which the NHS provides efficient services, including:
  — cost per unit of care/outcome
  — productivity of capital estate
  — labour productivity

- **Patient/carer experience**
  Patient/carer perceptions on the delivery of services, including:
  — responsiveness to individual needs and preferences
  — the skill care and continuity of service provision

— the physical environment; the organisation and courtesy of administrative arrangements

- **Health outcomes of NHS care**
  NHS success in using its resources to:
  — reduce levels of risk factors
  — reduce levels of disease, impairment and complications of treatment
  — improve quality of life for patients and carers
  — reduce premature deaths

Source: DOH, 1998.

References

Acheson, D. (1998) *Independent Inquiry into Inequalities in Health*. Report. The Stationery Office, London.

Black, D. (1980) Inequalities in health. In: *Inequalities in Health and the Health Divide*, (eds P. Townsend & N. Davidson). Penguin, London.

BMA (1996) *Core Services – Taking the Initiative*. General Practitioners Committee, British Medical Association, London.

Cadbury, A. (1992) *Aspects of Corporate Governance* (The Cadbury Report). Gee & Co., London.

Coffey, T., Boersma, G., Smith, L. & Wallace, P. (eds) (1999) *Visions of Primary Care*. New Health Network, Kings Fund, London.

CPT (1991) *Report to the UK Government. Visit to the UK, 1990*. The European Committee for the Prevention of Torture.

CPT (1996) *Report to the UK Government. Visit to the UK, 1994*. The European Committee for the Prevention of Torture.

DOH (1998) *A First Class Service – Quality in the New NHS*. Department of Health, London.

DOH (1999a) *National Service Framework for Mental Health – Modern Standards and Service Models*. Department of Health, London.

DOH (1999b) *The Future Organisation of Prison Health Care*. Report by the Joint Prison Service and National Health Service Executive Working Group. Department of Health, London.

DOH (2000a) *Nursing in Prisons*. Report by the Joint Prison Service and National Health Service Executive Working Group. Department of Health, London.

DOH (2000b) *Prison Handbook*. Prison Health Policy Unit and Task Force, Department of Health, London.

DOH (2000c) *Quality and Performance in the NHS: NHS Performance Indicators 1998/99*. Department of Health, London.

DOH (2000d) *The NHS Plan: A Plan for Investment – A Plan for Reform*. Cm 4818-I. The Stationery Office, London.

Dowling, A. (1983) *Health for a Change – the Provision of Preventive Health Care in Pregnancy and Early Childhood*. Child Poverty Action Group/National Extension College,

Greenbury, R. (1995) *Directors' Remuneration* (The Greenbury Report). Gee & Co., London.

Griffiths, J. (1991) Lessons in class. *Health Service Journal*, 22 August, pp. 20–21.

Hampel, R. (1998) *The Report of the Committee on Corporate Governance* (The Hampel Report). Gee & Co., London.

Hasler, J. (1993) The primary health care team – history and contractual farces. In: *Change and Teamwork in Primary Care*, (ed. M. Pringle). BMJ Publishing, London.

HMCIP (1994) *Report on HMP Leeds 20–24 June 1994*. HM Chief Inspector of Prisons, Home Office, London.

HMCIP (2001) *Patient or Prisoner? A Thematic Report on Prison Health Care*. HM Chief Inspector of Prisons, Home Office, London.

HMIP (1996) *Patient or Prisoner? A New Strategy for Health Care in Prisons*. Discussion paper. HM Inspectorate of Prisons, London.

Home Office (2000) *Prison Statistics: England and Wales 1999*. Cm 4805. The Stationery Office, London.

Kennedy, C. (1993) *Guide to the Management Gurus*. Century Business, London.

Lilley, R. (1999) *The PCG Toolkit – A Workbook for the Health Service and Primary Care Team*, 2nd edn. Radcliffe Medical Press, Oxford.

Meads, E. (ed.) (1996) *A Primary Care-Led NHS – Putting it into Practice*. Churchill Livingstone, Edinburgh.

Sines, D. (2001) *Community Healthcare Nursing*, 2nd edn, ch.1. Blackwell Science Ltd, Oxford.

Singleton, N. (1998) *Psychiatric Morbidity among Prisoners in England and Wales*. Office of National Statistics, The Stationery Office, London.

Stevens, A., Marshall, T. & Simpson, S. (2000) *Toolkit for Health Care Needs Assessment in Prisons – Health Care in Prisons: A Health Care Needs Assessment*. University of Birmingham, Birmingham.

Whitehead, M. (1992) The health divide. In: *Inequalities in Health and The Health Divide*, (eds P. Townsend & N. Davidson). Penguin, London.

Wilson, H. (1976) *The Governance of Britain*. Weidenfeld and Nicolson, London.

van Zwanenberg, T. & Harrison, J. (eds) (2000) *Clinical Governance in Primary Care*. Radcliffe Medical Press, Abingdon.

10 A Reflective View

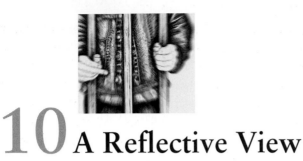

STEPHEN GANNON

Stephen Gannon's chapter is appropriately placed at the end of this book. Stephen provides honest and open views that are often considered to be 'alternative' by some, and which challenge traditional thinking. Stephen has developed a respect among many of his colleagues that helped earn him an MBE in 2000.

Having reached this last chapter, the reader will have learned a number of important things about prison nursing:

- prison nursing is unique
- prison nursing is an exciting professional challenge
- prison nursing is for the bold and forward-thinking nurse who is not afraid of rising to the challenge.

The opportunity to look back on so many years of service, both at junior and senior levels, is not given to many of us, and it is wonderful to have the means now to reflect openly on issues in a way not afforded to most prison nurses.

Since my own days as a prison nurse I have had the chance to go back into prisons, in a consultancy capacity, at three different establishments. This has been difficult and demanding, but it has enabled me to top up my personal experiences with a view from a new perspective. I have been able to see healthcare staff from the position of an outsider, joining the workforce on a temporary basis. Few working groups welcome a stranger who is sent in with the express remit of bringing about change (see Chapter 4, 'Understanding and Changing the Dynamics of the Prison Culture'). In any organisation most staff go to work wanting to do a good job, and they can find it hard to come to terms with senior management introducing someone outside the organisation to 'sort things out'.

Experience-fed practice as opposed to evidence-based practice is a rather dated concept in these days of tightly referenced research findings, and no two prison nurses would describe their role in identical terms. This chapter offers a personal view, hewn from my own experience. I do not seek to convert anyone to my own ideas, as I believe that we as individuals and the service as a whole are so much richer for our personal and collective differences.

Starting point

I was one of ten new nurses starting in prison healthcare, and was lucky enough to undergo a two-week course organised and run by two specialist training governors who came to London from their base at Newbold Revel, the Prison Service training establishment near Rugby.

These governors delivered a valuable syllabus covering the issues involved in effective prison healthcare. These included security awareness, control and restraint, radio procedures and adjudication systems, and there was a valuable opportunity to learn through roleplay. This is known within the prison service as a 'jailcraft course', and I was glad to have this exposure to real issues in prison life. It is a matter of some sadness to me that other nurses either have not had this opportunity, or get it later than they should. This is a major concern, and one that is raised regularly in HM Chief Inspector of Prisons reports. Basic induction training should be a prerequisite for all nurses new to prison life.

Both custodial and health staff care for prisoners, and there is often no clear demarcation. Nurses do not have exclusive rights to care for a prisoner while prison officers have a clear duty of care. There are many examples of considerate compassion shown daily by prison officers that would match that of our best nurses. At the same time, prison officers do not have an exclusive claim on security issues. There is a clear expectation that prison nursing must maintain safety and security as a responsibility to the general public, and this is fully endorsed by the NMC. There are some prison nurses who pay inappropriate attention to their security responsibilities, and who do not understand, or choose to ignore, the delicate balance between custody and care. Such carers would do well to reflect on the nursing code of conduct and the nature of caring.

Patient or prisoner?

The patient–prisoner context requires examination. The duality was prominently expressed by Her Majesty's Chief Inspector of Prisons in *Patient or Prisoner?* (HMCIP, 2001), and has had a profound effect in raising the issue of prisoners' healthcare to the top of the custodial agenda. The Chief Inspector has been extremely effective in gaining media coverage, which has opened up the debate outside the prison service. The discussion document *Patient or Prisoner?* (HMIP, 1996) also stimulated much debate and discussion at all levels in the service, suggesting new and workable partnership arrangements with local NHS providers.

It was clear that if the status quo remained unchallenged, the healthcare service for prisoners would continue to come a poor second to security, and that governors would continue to provide only the best healthcare service they could afford, recognising that it was not an organisational imperative. A prison governor must deliver core organisational targets – for example the number of escapes and assaults – in preference to healthcare targets.

The business infrastructure of a prison – its internal bureaucracy and financial arrangements – is primarily aimed at serving the courts. The prison service has a clear statutory responsibility for custody and rehabilitation, but until the prison service can engage the NHS in its statutory responsibility towards inmates as patients, prisons will continue to fail their prisoners. The NHS must be persuaded that each pound spent on a contained and engaged prisoner is almost always more effectively and efficiently spent than it would be if spent on that prisoner when back in the community. It is a social injustice that a person becomes disenfranchised in relation to healthcare simply by virtue of becoming a prisoner. The punishment should be the deprivation of personal freedom, not the deprivation of the right of access to the full state healthcare system. Perpetuating a second-class prison healthcare system is grossly unjust.

Prison and NHS partnership

The Future Organisation of Prison Health Care (DOH, 1999a) called for a reappraisal of healthcare delivery in prisons. It did not give a definitive statement, or a preferred model. There were clearly enormous difficulties in appeasing two major competitors for funding, the Home Office and the Department of Health. The report went for the middle ground – partnership, and as in many partnerships each partner has its own view about its responsibilities. 'Partnership' is a subjective term, and bespeaks the language of a populist administration. It would have been much more useful if legislators were clearer in their definitions of terms such as 'responsibility' and 'accountability'.

The medical model

The report did recognise the over-reliance on the medical model of management (paragraph 18) and the underdeveloped role of nurses (paragraph 20). It did not comment on the medical control model contained in Standing Order 13 (a prison rule) that has consistently failed to generate the momentum for change. This has been very apparent to HM Chief Inspector of Prisons. The senior medical officer in a prison had total authority over all healthcare matters and, being employed by the prison, was performance-managed by the prison governor. The report recommended a programme of change, including the health needs analysis of prisoners and the formation of the Prison Health Task Force and the Prison Health Policy Unit. It also identified a range of actions to address specific weaknesses, most notable of which was the issue of prisoners with mental health problems.

It is useful to note some continuity in government policy. Hard on the heels of *The Future Organisation of Prison Health Care* in July 2000, *The NHS Plan* (DOH, 2000b) further defined and specified policies planned to be in place by April 2004. The *National Service Framework – Mental Health* (DOH, 1999b) also mentions prisoners, particularly in relation to reducing suicides.

There are links developing between prisons and local NHS providers, and examples of co-operation and partnership are now more common and growing. An opportunity should be given to the Commission for Health Improvement to inspect a prison and measure local NHS trust performance against the existing national service framework policy. This would be a useful exercise and would set a target for future services to aim for.

Prisoners now have the right to consult with a doctor within 24 hours of demand, which compares favourably with proposal that all citizens be able to consult their GP within 48 hours by 2004 (DOH, 2000b); in this instance prisoners fare better than the general public. While not being complacent about some underachieving areas in prison primary care, especially in preventative health promotion activities such as smoking cessation, we can say that there are clear improvements in many areas.

Mental health and patient care in prisons

By far the most pressing clinical condition in prisons is mental illness (Singleton, 1998). Estimates of mentally ill prisoners range from 40% to 70% of the total prison population, and similar estimates for the remand population are even vaguer. When combined with the estimates for prisoners involved with substance abuse this figure rises to around 90%. The assessment tools used to reach these figures tend to be quite rudimentary. Form F2069, a healthcare assessment questionnaire, is completed at all new receptions; page three of this form asks only a few simple questions about mental health history.

The most interesting predictors of potential mental problems tend to be hard to identify. Those prisoners most at risk of serious suicidal intent are not identified by the current documentation system (F2052SH), while most serious self-harming incidents follow hard on the heels of 'fresh' imprisonment. In the light of this knowledge, newly received prisoners should be particularly sensitively supervised for a period of at least two weeks, with higher than normal staffing ratios, and the prison should adopt an active intervention strategy rather than just responding passively. The beginning of internment or a change of prison often creates a setting in which prisoners can become wracked by ugly reflection, especially when they are encouraged to confront their criminal lifestyle isolated behind bars. This may be their first time for lucid reflection on a miserable life without the distractions and disguise of drink and drugs. It is at this point in a sentence where sensitive handling and skilled care from a nurse is most needed.

Through the creation of the Safer Prisons Unit, the prison service is currently in the process of creating a refreshing system-wide approach to the care of the self-harmer. This group is piloting innovative approaches in several prisons, introducing for example safer cell design and listener suites. This underlines the awareness that prison professionals must be ready with new skills and resources as these come on line.

If we accept that many prisoners have mental health problems, it follows that their care requirements are often extremely challenging. The 1999 publication *The Future Organisation of Prison Health Care* (DOH, 1999a) recommends that secondary care continues to be the responsibility of the NHS, ensuring that community mental health services reach into prisons and that mentally ill offenders who require hospital care are adequately provided for. It is crucially important in the new partnership arrangements with the NHS that this element of the service retains its priority status.

Nursing in Prisons

Nursing in Prisons, published in October 2000 (DOH, 2000a), also addresses the care of mentally ill people in prisons and recommends solutions. Another important reference is the Health Advisory Committee (HAC) for the prison service's report *The Provision of Mental Health Care in Prisons* (Home Office, 1997). Although the problem has been highlighted, it has not yet been considered politically important enough to resource. Again, much hope is placed on the new partnership arrangements with the NHS. Local NHS community mental health teams (CMHTs) should as a matter of course be taking part in ward rounds and case reviews inside the prison, and be committing themselves to healthcare assessments as part of new reception procedures. They should also be encouraged to offer support to wing-based staff to care for prisoners on residential landings, and should become part of the prison's suicide prevention committee.

False perceptions

The prison service has not had the resources to fund inpatient services to a level concomitant with its own definition of healthcare standards or to that of the NHS. This is changing, however, as political pressure and media attention demand that equity and individuals' rights are adhered to. The Chief Inspector's team assesses practice against the *Health Care Standards for Prisoners in England and Wales* (HM Prison Service, 1994). These nine standards range from first reception into prisons through to the safe storage and administration of medication. The prison service has taken account of these standards, yet recently issued a similar but briefer set (HM Prison Service, 2000) that differs significantly in its content. Which is the preferred set? Are the original standards still pertinent? There is an urgent need for a baseline standard that identifies resource requirements against outcomes. NHS regions have clear guidelines when they are designing secure services for the mentally ill; among other issues these guidelines specify acceptable staff-to-patient ratios. Prisons within equivalent NHS regional boundaries should be similarly specific in allocating ring-fenced resources. This raises the concern that we should not be constructing parallel systems, but it would be quite appropriate to recommend that, if the current strategy of keeping mentally ill people in prisons remains unchallenged, there should at the very least be adequate resourcing of the service.

The NHS provides six beds per 1000 population. The prison service provides 28. Even allowing for the high rates of morbidity in the prison service this a significant difference (Marshall, 1999). Mental health patients occupy the majority (75%) of beds in prison healthcare centres (Reed & Lyne, 2000).

False perceptions

The care of mentally ill prisoners is a recurrent problem. More specifically, it is the inpatient care of mentally ill prisoners that is of regular concern. I have already indicated that the current medical model is obsolete, and that the community care model is the only practical model for the future. Where prisons are concerned, residential wings are the community. If all care were on the wings, why not call in a crisis intervention team from the NHS in the event of a psychiatric emergency? If it is felt that inpatient care is necessary, then it should be arranged in the same manner as if the emergency had happened in the wider community. At worst, prisons could retain a 72-hour crisis response centre, giving enough time to refer patients to NHS agencies and construct a wing-based care plan with visiting community mental healthcare teams, or a court order supporting movement to an NHS unit. A daycare area could be attached to this crisis centre, where prisoners could be supported on residential landings offering self-help skills; this could perhaps be maintained by attendance at the day centre following discharge from a period of crisis. The day centre could become the new focus of activity in prison healthcare.

There is a real opportunity to be grasped in challenging the traditional model and moving to a community-based care model. As I have indicated, NHS CMHT inreach teams should feature prominently in such a model, which should also value the skills of prison officers on residential landings and place the prisoner at the centre of the efforts being made to improve the situation. The revision of the current Mental Health Act of 1983 came out as a White Paper in December 2000 (DOH & Home Office, 2000). Although there is no specific proposal to widen the Act to cover the treatment of mentally ill people in prisons, the thin end of a reform wedge is introduced in Part 1, paragraphs 4.11 and 4.12, which refer to 'specialist assessment' and, more worryingly, 'an appropriate environment, which could be in a hospital, or a dedicated section of a prison'.

Society should expect people to receive mental health care in appropriately resourced facilities with the resources of a truly multi-disciplinary team. A prison is a fundamentally unhealthy place in which to explore a prisoner's mental health issues, and there needs to be considerable debate about the implications of the care and management of mentally ill prisoners if we are to legitimise the mental health assessment process while they are in the physical confines of a prison. Every patient in a hospital can expect to have full access to nurses and doctors, yet prisoners are locked up for at least 12 out of every 24 hours. Where does the proposed assessment period begin and end? Can we truly assess someone who is locked behind his or her cell door for such lengthy periods? Surely the 'appropriate place' remains a hospital. We should not easily tolerate an erosion of this principle without the most exacting scrutiny of the resources to be committed to a proposed alternative.

There should be an urgent revision by the judiciary of the current practice of remanding people to prisons for psychiatric reports. It is a wrong that people who appear obviously mentally ill – to a degree that makes it necessary to seek such a report – are sent to prisons, which are not resourced, to carry out the process. This too is a political issue that needs addressing, and staff are to be complimented on their efforts to provide a service in the current climate.

In October 2000 newly introduced European human rights legislation enabled prisoners to seek redress if they feel that they have been unable to access mental healthcare systems equivalent to those available if they had they not been detained in prison. It cannot be long before somebody challenges their right to be in a more appropriate environment than a prison.

Healthcare staffing issues

Carer support and clinical supervision have been very patchy across the prison service. In my view all registered nurses working in prisons should be 'retained' by the local NHS trust and 'outposted' to the prison. By rejoining local NHS trusts, prison nurses will benefit from the protective maturity of an appropriately-resourced 'parent' organisation that can afford to support clinical supervision and governance, and offer training and educational updating. This may include a form of professional relief, where nurses can temporarily work in A&E or an acute psychiatric unit for a few weeks without altering their employment conditions, but can update and refresh their professional skills. Conversely, nurses in local acute psychiatric units may wish to experience the prison system in order to broaden their knowledge. Nobody should be forced along this route, however; it must remain the desire of the individual nurse and the gift of the employer. Crucially, it should never be used to plug short-term gaps in the NHS or within the prison.

I would never suggest that prison nursing is automatically de-skilling or draining; to some it is an area rich with opportunity and challenge. Registered nurses will be in short supply for many years to come, and the UKCC/NMC statistics demonstrate a bulge of nurses coming up to retirement. This sets a significant challenge for those who are responsible for the recruitment of staff over the next decade. It also sets a challenge for senior healthcare managers to make the service attractive and rewarding enough to attract the dynamic type of nurse the service needs. We must embrace the full range of skills involved in patient/prisoner care. The Royal College of Nursing, during its annual general meeting in October 2000, opened up the possibility of healthcare assistants, having attained a defined level of competence, joining its membership in some form. It could be suggested that prison officers' skills might fall within such a structure.

Prison officers can now be considered for healthcare officer training via the competence framework of the NVQ structure, and in the autumn of 2001 an NVQ in custodial care was introduced. In the interim period, any prison officer training should aim to embrace healthcare. Any courses now being constructed would do well to use the UKCC document of November 1999, *Nursing in Secure Environments* (UKCC & University of Central Lancashire, 1999), which contains many of the competences identified to date. There are many dedicated and professional prison officers in the service who may wish to develop their skills and competences in a healthcare setting. The Director-General of the prison service has made statements committing officers to learning mental health skills. These skills are transferable to residential landings and will assist officers to develop their careers. If officers wish to work in healthcare centres it will assist their hard-pressed nursing colleagues who are in such short supply. Officer colleagues, with the right training opportunities, have consistently proved that they make excellent members of the healthcare team.

The benefit of an adequately resourced healthcare centre is that nurses can be used to their full potential: nurse-run clinics and nurse prescribing are just two examples. This is exactly what was recognised in the *Nursing in Prisons* report (DOH, 2000a).

Staff values and attitudes

Considering officers for placement in healthcare settings raises another question. How do we select people with an acceptable value and attitude set? I believe that the prison service works hard to recruit appropriately through its officer selection procedures, which deliberately focus on personal attitudes. We need to ensure that the same care is taken in employing nurses. Only people with a strong and robust nursing value set should be employed, people who understand that kindness is not about weakness and can defend that principle in an articulate manner. Socially closed institutions, such as mental hospitals and prisons, sometimes attract people with personal needs incompatible with an acceptable value system.

How a prisoner is addressed is a good example of new attitudes. There is nothing more individual than a person's name. The way you are addressed can make all the difference to how you feel about yourself, and it is in this area that staff from outside the prison often set an example to staff who have traditionally worked in an environment that tends to be rather regimented and has lost some of the empathy and sensitivity that it should have.

Prison nursing – is it a specialism?

One way to resist the assimilation of poor habits is to make it clear what professional expectations are being aimed for. Ask any prison nurse if they think that they are a defined speciality in the family of nursing, and they will say yes. Ask them to expand on that, to tell you what standards they work to, and they will often be lost. Is it the actual interventions that are special, or is it the environment in which they are practised that is unique? At the last three annual RCN prison nurse conferences of the twentieth century, prison nurses have been challenged to define their area of speciality (see Chapter 1, 'The Context of Prison Nursing'). At conferences we all exude enthusiasm and interest, yet on returning to everyday clinical practice we are inevitably subsumed and overwhelmed by the daily grind. The RCN forum commissioned a project to define prison nursing, which was published in the autumn of 2001 (RCN, 2001). One only has to look at nurses working in high security hospitals to understand that there is a clear security function; the purist argument that supports no security responsibility lacks the insight of the rich skill base to be found in balancing the need to maintain a safe and secure environment while promoting high standards of nursing care. It is this delicate balance that challenges and defines the nurse working in the prison environment.

No limits

Prison healthcare is fascinating, and not for the fainthearted. The potential for professional development is boundless. Every aspect of the NHS agenda is relevant to the prison service, and the NHS is on the cusp of a new relationship with prisons that will be much more important and productive for all our citizens than it has been in the past. It is a new and socially inclusive paradigm.

I recall an NHS experiment some years ago in which nurses managed and developed their own strategic decisions about how beds should be allocated. Groups of nurses or 'nursing development units' admitted and discharged to their own wards. Prison healthcare centres would be the ideal environment for the re-establishment of this model, in which nurses would prepare and present the case for such an experiment. With the movement of NHS inreach teams from local trusts into prisons there is a real opportunity for prison nursing to become a prestigious nursing care area, managed and led by nurses.

Proposals for positive change

(1) All new entrants into the prison healthcare workforce should take part in a common induction programme of no less than two weeks; this should be issued as a prison service instruction to all prisons.
(2) Staff taking different routes into the prison healthcare environment should have a common uniform.

(3)   National service framework targets should be measured by the Commission for Health Improvement.

(4)   Information technology resources consisting of NHS links into the prison and internal local area networks should urgently be established. The software should contain elements of NHS Direct and electronic prescribing. The photograph taken of each prisoner during current reception procedures should be incorporated into the NHS healthcare system.

(5)   Redefine the IMR. With the rapid development in custody nurses being used in police stations, this document would ideally originate at the initial point of detention and follow the detained person throughout the system (similar to the existing PER). This would make reception healthcare screening richer in content. The document should be renamed the Integrated Healthcare Record. Each healthcare profession should make records only in this common document.

(6)   All new receptions, for the high risk period of four weeks, should be located in residential areas with higher than average staffing ratios, including visiting community mental healthcare teams. An active intervention strategy should be developed; with the high suicide rate in our prisons passive regimes are no longer acceptable.

(7)   The Task Force Policy Unit should clarify and unify the two current sets of healthcare standards, and include definitions of inputs and resources as well as outputs and standards.

(8)   HCC inpatient beds should be closed. It is not a function of a prison to be an NHS hospital. The creation of a daycare centre would become the focal point of the prison's healthcare activity. If a crisis suite is retained, it should close during the day while all of the staff and any patients are employed in the day centre. This proposal would do more than any other single recommendation to create a cultural change.

(9)   Every prison should have a dedicated NHS community mental health inreach team which shadows prisoners from reception through to discharge.

(10) There should be a judicial review of the current practice of remanding mentally ill people to prisons for reports.

(11) The Mental Health Act White Paper (DOH & Home Office, 2000) suggestion to create dedicated assessment areas in prisons should be robustly debated, as it is a departure from previous mental health policy and was not proposed in the preceding Green Paper.

(12) Nurses employed in prisons should become 'subsets' of local NHS trusts.

(13) The new Nursing and Midwifery Council (previously the UKCC) should develop a code of ethics specifically for nurses working in prisons.

(14) Prison service healthcare policy units should clarify the practice of unregistered healthcare officers being allocated clinical roles that are identical with those of registered nurses.

References

DOH (1999a) *The Future Organisation of Prison Health Care*. Report by the Joint Prison Service and National Health Service Executive Working Group. Department of Health, London.

DOH (1999b) *National Service Framework – Mental Health*. Report by the Joint Prison Service and National Health Service Executive Working Group. Department of Health, London.

DOH (2000a) *Nursing in Prisons*. Report by the Joint Prison Service and National Health Service Executive Working Group. Department of Health, London.

DOH (2000b) *The NHS Plan: A Plan for Investment – A Plan for Reform*. Cm 4818-I. The Stationery Office, London.

DOH & Home Office (2000) *Reforming the Mental Health Act*. Cm 5016-I & II. The Stationery Office, London.

HMCIP (2001) *Patient or Prisoner? A Thematic Report on Prison Health Care*. HM Chief Inspector of Prisons, Home Office, London.

HMIP (1996) *Patient or Prisoner? A New Strategy for Health Care in Prisons*. Discussion paper. HM Inspectorate of Prisons, London.

Home Office (1997) *The Provision of Mental Health Care in Prisons*. Health Advisory Committee for the Prison Service in England and Wales, London.

RCN (2001) *Caring for Prisoners*. Royal College of Nursing, London.

Reed, J. & Lyne, M. (2000) Inpatient care of mentally ill people in prisons: results of a year's programme of semi-structured inspections. *British Medical Journal*, **320**, 1031–4.

Singleton, N. (1998) *Psychiatric Morbidity among Prisoners in England and Wales*. Office of National Statistics, The Stationery Office, London.

UKCC & University of Central Lancashire (1999) *Nursing in Secure Environments*. United Kingdom Central Council for Nursing, Midwifery and Health Visiting, London.

Index

aftercare, 10
aggression, 54
AIDS/HIV, 107
alcohol, 33, 144
Armley Prison (Leeds)
  clinical governance
    framework and, 151–5
  Committee for the
    Prevention of Torture
    (CPT) report, 137
  governor's experience,
    135–76
  health needs assessment,
    149–50
  healthcare staff and centre,
    136, 138–9, 141–2, 146,
    150, 152, 167
  HM Chief Inspector of
    Prisons reports, 138, 139
  industrial relations, 135,
    169–70
  medical staff problems,
    136, 139–40, 148, 156,
    157
  office management, 167
  overcrowding, 136–7
  reception process, 136,
    139, 148, 169–70
Ashworth Hospital, 88
attitudes, 53–5, 186

babies in prison, 96, 107,
  115–16
beds, numbers of, 149, 174
behavioural theories of
  learning, 68, 69–70
benzodiazepines, 161
Bland, Tony, 105
body searches, 22

Bolam test, 103
bullying, 49

Canada, 81–2
care
  aftercare, 10
  care and programme
    management, 7
  duty of, 100–102, 103, 179
  local authority care, 114
  national vocational
    qualifications (NVQs),
    88
  negligence, 99–100, 102,
    103
  standards of, 102–3
career progression, 38–9
categories of prisons, 2–3
challenges, 15, 20–21, 43
change, 178–9
  attitudes, 54–5
  cultural, 55–6
  quality healthcare, 119–21
  role of nurse in prison and,
    21–2, 24–5, 187–9
children
  babies in prison, 96, 107,
    115–16
  of prisoners, 145
  sexual offences against,
    108–10
  young offenders, 5–6,
    114–15
client group, 4–5, 17–18, 33,
  143, 172, 174, 180
clinical governance, 128, 129,
  133–4, 151–5
clinical practice, 7
clinics, nurse-led, 17

cognitive learning, 68, 69
Commission for Health
  Improvement (CHI), 100
Committee for the Prevention
  of Torture (CPT), 137
communication, 16–17
Community Justice National
  Training Organisation
  (NTO), 86, 87–8
comparative needs, 9
competences, 75–7, 78–94
compliance, 50, 51
conditions of service, 39–40
confidentiality, 97, 110–113,
  125
conflict, 49–50
conformity, 50, 51
conjugal visits, 108
consent, 97
  to disclosure of confidential
    information, 111
context of prison nursing,
  1–13
control, culture and, 47–50
culture, 45–57, 126, 127
  attitudes, 53–5, 186
  compliance and conformity,
    50, 51
  control and, 47–50
  dynamics of change, 55–6
  groups, 46, 47, 51–2
  of learning, 60–61
  meaning of, 46–7
  role and, 52–3
  sanctions, 46
  socialisation, 50–55
Custodial Care National
  Training Organisation
  (NTO), 36, 86–7, 91

data protection, 113
degrading treatment, 105, 106, 137
detention centres, 6
discrimination, prohibition of, 110
diversion to mental hospitals, 167
doctors
　General Practitioners (GPs), 163, 165
　medical staff problems in Armley Prison (Leeds), 136, 139–40, 148, 156, 157
　primary care, 163
　primary care contacts, 149–50
　prison reception process, 136, 139, 148, 169–70
drugs
　dependence, 33
　treatment centre, 150
duty of care, 100–102, 103

education and training, 12, 36–8, 40, 58–73, 75–94, 126
　competences, 75–7, 78–94
　culture of learning, 60–61
　evidence-based practice, 72–3
　learning styles, 71–2
　learning theories, 68–71
　lifelong learning, 58, 59–60
　maintenance of registration, 61–8
　meeting patients' needs, 78
　professional profile, 63–6
　reflection, 66–8
　secure environments project, 78, 88–91
　study days, 61–3
emergencies, psychiatric, 184
empowerment, 11, 116
environment, healthy, 9–10, 11, 131–4
ethnic minorities, 22, 143
European Committee for the Prevention of Torture (CPT), 137
European Convention of Human Rights, 104–10
evidence-based practice, 72–3
expectations, 48, 52

experiential learning, 68, 71
expressed needs, 9

facilitation of health-enhancing activities, 11
fair trial right, 106–7
family life, 144–6
　conjugal visits, 108
　respect for, 107
　right to marry, 110
felt needs, 8

General Practitioners (GPs), 163, 165
government, 154
　health policies
　　development, 29–32, 181
　　development of competences, 78–88
　　influencing, 12
groups
　culture and, 46, 47, 51–2
　teamwork, 16–17, 35–6

health assessment, 4–5
health authorities,
　performance indicators, 160
healthcare officers, 33–4, 39, 97, 144, 162, 185–6
health centres, 164
health improvement
　healthy environment, 9–10, 11, 131–4
　performance indicators, 161, 175–6
　plans for (HImP), 122, 150
health indicators, 162, 175–6
health needs, 8–9, 33, 78, 126
　assessment of, 12, 33, 149–50
health policies
　development, 29–32, 181
　development of competences, 78–88
　influencing, 12
healthy environment, 9–10, 11, 131–4
heart attacks, 160
Her Majesty's Chief Inspector of Prisons, 4, 118, 127, 131, 138
higher level of practice pilot standard (HLP), 85–6
high security prisons, 2–3

historical background of healthcare in prison, 27–9
HIV, 107
hospitals
　diversion to mental hospitals, 167
　performance indicators, 160
　pressures on, 164–5
Howard, John, 28
human rights issues, 104–10

industrial relations, 135, 169–70
inequalities in health, 142–4, 172–3
inhuman treatment, 105, 106, 137
isolation, 50

judgements, 19, 49

Kray, Reggie, 106

Lancaster Farms (young offender institution), 6
language difficulties, 22
leadership, 6, 18–19, 40–43
learning
　behavioural theories, 68, 69–70
　cognitive learning, 68, 69
　culture of, 60–61
　evidence-based practice, 72–3
　experiential, 68, 71
　factors affecting, 72
　lifelong learning, 58, 59–60
　meeting objectives, 68–71
　social theories, 68, 70–71
　styles, 71–2
legal issues, 96–116
　confidentiality, 97, 110–113, 125
　data protection, 113
　duty of care, 100–102, 103
　human rights issues, 104–10
　negligence, 99–100, 102, 103
　regulation of nursing profession, 98–9
　standards of care, 102–3
　young offenders, 114–15
life, right to, 105

local authority care, 114

management
    care and programme
        management, 7
    medical model, 181
    National Health Service
        (NHS), 127, 154
    practice managers, 164
    as profession, 153–4
    see also leadership
marriage
    conjugal visits, 108
    right to marry, 110
medical model, 181
medical records, 107, 111–12
medical treatment, obligations
    to provide, 105, 106
men in prison, 5, 33, 145
    suicide, 101–2, 143–4, 159,
        182
mental health problems, 10,
        33, 102, 130, 145,
        167–8, 181–5
    confidentiality and, 112
    diversion to mental
        hospitals, 167
    false perceptions, 183–5
    NHS and, 158, 168
    obligations to provide
        medical treatment for
        patients, 106
    psychiatric emergencies,
        184
    suicide, 101–2, 143–4, 159,
        182
mothers and babies, 96, 107,
        115–16

names, 186
National Health Service (NHS)
    formation, 153
    management, 127, 154
    mental health problems
        and, 158, 168
    national service
        frameworks, 158–9
    partnership arrangements
        with, 21–2, 24, 30,
        118–19, 121, 141, 146–
        8, 180–181
    performance assessment,
        156–7
    performance indicators,
        159–62, 175–6

plan for future of, 128–31
National Training Organisa-
    tions (NTOs), 36, 86–8,
    91
national vocational qualifica-
    tions (NVQs), 36, 37, 88,
    92
needs
    health needs, 8–9, 33, 78,
        126
    assessment of, 12, 33,
        149–50
    security needs of prison, 16,
        24, 46–7, 179
negligence, 99–100, 102, 103
normative needs, 8
nurse-led clinics, 17
Nursing and Midwifery
    Council (NMC), vi, 3,
        20, 97, 99, 124, 179
    and PREP, 55
    code of practice, 54, 123–4
    higher level of practice pilot
        standard (HLP), 85–6
    pre-registration standards,
        84–5
    professional profile, 64
    quality healthcare and,
        123–5
    registration, 61–4, 84–5
    regulation of nursing
        profession, 99

occupational standards
    (competences), 75–7,
    78–94
open prisons, 3
overcrowding, 136–7

partnership arrangements
    with NHS, 21–2, 24, 30,
        118–19, 121, 141, 146–8,
        180–181
patients, 154–5
    client group, 4–5, 17–18,
        33, 143, 172, 174, 180
    confidentiality, 97,
        110–113, 125
    duty of care to, 100–102,
        103, 179
    health assessment, 4–5
    health needs, 8–9, 33, 78,
        126
    assessment of, 12, 33,
        149–50

nurse-patient relationships,
    15–17, 126
    quality healthcare for,
        118–34
    seeking views from, 121–2
    see also mental health
        problems
performance assessment,
    156–7
performance indicators,
    159–62, 175–6
persistent vegetative state
    (PVS), 105
persuasion, 55
portfolios, 64
power, 49
practice managers, 164
practice nurses, 163
prevention of ill health, 9–11
primary care, 163–7
    contacts, 149–50
    groups/trusts, 165–6
    meaning of, 166
    NHS national service
        frameworks, 158–9
    prospects for, 166–7
prison categories, 2–3
prison culture see culture
prison governor, view of
    healthcare in prison,
    135–76
Prison Health Policy Unit and
    Task Force (PHPU/TF),
    30, 146, 147–8
prison nurses, 33–5
    career progression, 38–9
    challenges for, 15, 20–21,
        43
    change and, 21–2, 24–5,
        187–9
    current situation, 23–4
    getting it right, 19–20
    historical background,
        27–9
    nurse-patient relationships,
        15–17, 126
    primary care, 149–50
    quality healthcare and, 121,
        122–5, 126–8
    role of, 14–26
    social context, 2–6
    specialist practice, 6–7,
        186–7
    staffing issues, 185–6
        Armley Prison (Leeds),

136, 138–40, 141–2,
146, 148, 150, 152,
156, 157, 167
strategies, 35–9
terms and conditions of
service, 39–40
see also education and
training; legal issues; *and*
individual topics
prison officers
healthcare officers, 33–4,
39, 97, 144, 162, 185–6
industrial relations, 135,
169–70
prison culture and, 46, 47,
50–51, 52–3
private life, respect for, 107
professional duty of care,
100–102, 103, 179
professionalism, 16, 19–20
professional profile, 63–6
profiles, 63–6
psychiatric conditions *see*
mental health problems
punishment, prison as, 19–20,
48

quality healthcare, 118–34
health needs, 126
levers of change, 119–20
NHS plan, 128–31
prison nurses and, 121,
122–5, 126–8
professional
responsibilities, 126–8
progress with caution, 120
providing healthy
environment, 131–4
seeking views of patients,
121–2
structural changes,
120–121
UKCC and, 123–5

racial minorities, 22, 143
reception process, 136, 139,
148, 169–70

reflection, 66–8
registration, maintenance of,
61–8
regulation of nursing
profession, 98–9
rehabilitation, 48–9
relationships, nurse-patient,
15–17, 126
respect, 48
role, culture and, 52–3
role models, nurses as, 12

Sainsbury Centre for Mental
Health, 82–3
sanctions, 46
secure accommodation,
114–15
secure environments project,
78, 88–91
security needs of prison, 16,
24, 46–7, 179
sexual offences, 108–10
slopping out, 135
Smalley, Herbert, 28–9
social background
high security prisoners, 3
women prisoners, 4
social context of prison
nursing, 2–6
socialisation, 50–55
social learning theories, 68,
70–71
specialist practice, 6–7, 186–7
staffing issues, 33–5, 185–6
Armley Prison (Leeds), 136,
138–40, 141–2, 146,
148, 150, 152, 156,
157, 167
standards
of care, 102–3
occupational standards
(competences), 75–7,
78–94
strategies for prison nursing,
35–9
State Hospital for Scotland
(Carstairs), 83–4

study days, 61–3
suicide, 101–2, 143–4, 159,
182
supervision, 3, 19
teamwork, 16–17, 35–6
terms and conditions of
service, 39–40
textbook on prison nursing,
28–9
therapeutic approaches to
health and social well-
being, 12
torture, 105, 106
training *see* education and
training
trial, right to fair trial, 106–7
trust, position of, 108–10

United Kingdom Central
Council (UKCC), vi, 1,
2, 3, 6, 20, 37, 61, 63,
78, 80, 91, 97
pre-registration standards,
84–5
professional profile, 63–6
quality healthcare and,
123–5
regulation of nursing
profession, 98–9
University of Central
Lancashire, 88

values *see* culture
violence, 54
voluntary services, 48–9
vulnerable groups, 22–3
protection of, 10–11

women in prison, 4–5, 33
mothers and babies, 96,
107, 115–16
Women's Policy Unit, 5

young offenders, 5–6, 114–15